COMPLETE GUIDE TO CANCER NURSING

E D I T E D   B Y:

MARJORIE BEYERS, RN, PhD
Former Executive Director
National Commission on Nursing

JUNE WERNER, RN, MSN, CNAA
Chairman, Department of Nursing
Evanston Hospital

SUZANNE DURBURG, RN, BSN, MEd
Associate Chairman, Department of Nursing
Evanston Hospital

D0681728

MEDICAL ECONOMICS BOOKS
Oradell, New Jersey 07649

Library of Congress Cataloging in Publication Data

Main entry under title:

Complete guide to cancer nursing.

Includes bibliographical references and index.
1. Cancer—Nursing. I. Beyers, Majorie. II. Durburg,
Suzanne. III. Werner, June. [DNLM: 1. Neoplasms—
Nursing. WY 156 C737]
RC266.C65   1983   610.73'698   83-846
ISBN 0-87489-294-5

Cover design by Jerry Wilke

ISBN 0-87489-294-5

Medical Economics Company Inc.
Oradell, New Jersey 07649

Printed in the United States of America

To our cancer patients and their families

CONTENTS

PART I INTRODUCTION

PART II TREATMENT

PART III NURSING MANAGEMENT OF LONG-TERM CARE

PART IV SPECIAL CONSIDERATIONS

CONTRIBUTORS

Marjorie Beyers, RN, PhD, principal editor of this book, is also co-author, with Susan Dudas, of *The Clinical Practice of Medical-Surgical Nursing,* and with Carole Phillips, of *Nursing Management for Patient Care.* Dr. Beyers recently served as executive director of the National Commission on Nursing, a three-year study of nursing-related issues funded by the American Hospital Association, the Hospital Research and Educational Trust and the American Hospital Supplies Corporation.

June Werner, RN, MSN, CNAA, a co-editor of this book and author of Chapter 15, is chairman of the Department of Nursing, Evanston (Ill.) Hospital.

Suzanne Durburg, RN, BSN, MEd, also co-editor of this book and author of Chapters 1 and 13, is associate chairman of the Department of Nursing, Evanston Hospital.

Susan B. Anderson, RN, BSN, who wrote Chapter 5, is staff nurse, Kellogg Cancer Care Center, Evanston Hospital.

Julie Boyer, RD, author of Chapter 10, is clinical nutritional specialist, Evanston Hospital.

Jennifer Coates, RN, BSN, co-author of Chapter 7, is former staff nurse, Kellogg Cancer Care Center, Evanston Hospital.

Linda Dotson, RN, BSN, who wrote Chapter 2, is clinical director, Glenbrook (Ill.) Hospital.

Michelle McClanahan, RN, BS, co-author of Chapter 3 and author of Chapters 4, 6, and 12, is clinical director, Evanston Hospital.

Mary E. Mielnicki, RN, BSN, co-author of Chapter 3 and author of Chapters 8, 9, and 11, is staff nurse, Glenbrook (Ill.) Hospital.

Kimberly Raia, RN, MS, co-author of Chapter 7, is clinical coordinator, Kellogg Cancer Care Center, Evanston Hospital.

Patricia Wall, RN, who wrote Chapter 14, is former staff nurse, Evanston Hospital.

PREFACE

MARJORIE BEYERS, RN, PhD

This book was written to guide nurses in the care of patients during the different phases of cancer care. Written by staff nurses and others for their colleagues, the book is organized to provide essential and comprehensive information about oncology nursing in an easy-to-read style and format.

Two complementary forces stimulated the development of this book. The growing expertise of staff nurses at the Kellogg Cancer Care Center, located within the Evanston Hospital Corporation, was one force. The other was the increasing call upon these nurses to provide their colleagues in community hospitals with consultation and guidance in care of patients with cancer. Once the authors decided to commit their expertise to writing for use by their colleagues, the book grew from a set of guidelines to its current state.

Writing the book has been a professional accomplishment for the authors. Sharing one's clinical knowledge is a mark of the maturing professional. A book that consistently emphasizes the patient and family is an expression of professional values. Organizing a book that provides readers with information in a concise yet explanatory approach, is a challenge.

The patient-care information and nursing insights shared in this book represent a strong professional commitment on the part of both the authors and the hospital that provides the environment for their nursing practice. The material in this book was developed by nurses in practice and is currently used in patient care. All of the authors have had to clarify their own specialized nursing practice in communicating their knowledge. The result is a resource and a "colleague in print" for nurse generalists.

ACKNOWLEDGMENTS

The authors wish to thank our professional colleagues for contributing material used in the book. Staff nurses developed many of the Patient Care Guidelines presented here. Nurse clinicians formulated the Diagnostic Procedure Manual we used as a resource in Chapter 3.

We are also grateful to the many people who offered us guidance and reviewed our sections and chapters. In particular, we are indebted to Bonnie Meyers, RN, MSN, who graciously served as our expert reviewer for content, and to the following people and departments for their help and encouragement throughout the writing of the book:

KELLOGG CANCER CARE CENTER NURSING STAFF
Susan Boland, RN, MSN, Enterostomal Clinical Specialist, Evanston Hospital
Max Haid, MD, Physician, Medical Oncology, Evanston Hospital
Janardan Khandekar, MD, Director, Medical Oncology, Evanston Hospital
Peter Mudd, MSW, Executive Director, Jung Center, Evanston
Paul Perles, Librarian, Medical Library, Glenbrook Hospital
Edward F. Scanlon, MD, Chairman, Department of Surgery, Evanston Hospital
Stephen Sener, MD, Fellow, Oncology Surgery, Memorial Sloan-Kettering Cancer Center
Esther Tarnay, MSW, Director, Social Services, Evanston Hospital
Steven Tovian, PhD, Director of Psychosocial Counseling Services, Kellogg Cancer Care Center, Evanston Hospital

Finally, we wish to recognize Ann Larson for typing our many rough drafts and cheering us onward.

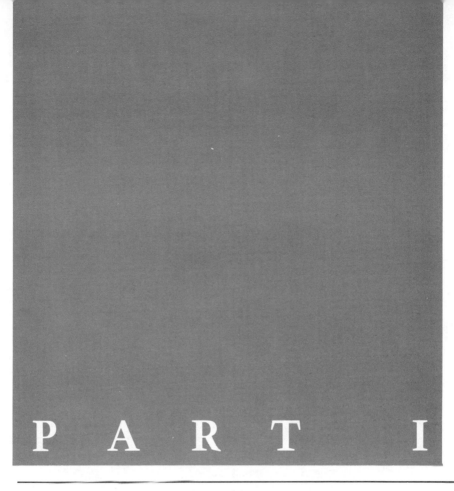

PART I

INTRODUCTION

1

THE NURSE IN CANCER CARE

SUZANNE DURBURG, RN, BSN, MEd

Fifty-six million Americans, or one in four, will have a cancer diagnosis at some point in their lifetime. The disease will affect two of every three families. In 1980, the American Cancer Society estimated that in the following year new cancers would be diagnosed in 805,000 people.[1] Of these, approximately 268,000 were expected to be alive in 1986. More than three million Americans alive today have a history of cancer, and of that number two million persons were initially diagnosed more than five years ago. Although the number of deaths from cancer per 100,000 population has increased since 1930, deaths from most major types of cancer generally are reaching a plateau and in some cancers are declining. This progress is the result of national efforts in research, prevention, and treatment directed at cancers of all kinds over the past years.

Centers dedicated to cancer treatment are at the cutting edge of research, treatment, and professional education; most cancer patients, however, are diagnosed and treated in whatever health-care facilities are in their communities. Nurses at these facilities are involved in all phases of care for cancer patients and their families. The various roles nurses play in such work are the subject of this book. This introductory chapter is intended to give an overview of cancer nursing.

Nursing has been defined as "helping people [sick or well] in the performance of those activities contributing to health, or its recovery [or to a peaceful death] that they would perform unaided if they had the necessary strength, will, or knowledge. It is likewise the unique contribution of nursing to help people be independent of such assistance as soon as possible."[2] In other words, the nurse is a professional who sustains patients in maintenance or restabilization of their health. Patients require nursing services at critical times when real or potential health problems or illness affect their daily living. As they do for patients in general, nurses provide care to cancer patients and their families in many different settings—in hospitals or homes, in physicians' offices, or in health-education primary-prevention programs.

Primary prevention

Encouraged by measurable successes that are due to the early diagnosis and treatment of cancer, health-care professionals have taken an aggressive approach toward primary prevention of cancer. Nurses in schools, cancer-prevention centers or programs, and in health-promotion programs in industry and elsewhere are actively educating the public about cancer. These health-education programs are intended to motivate people to modify life habits so they can control these factors—substances they eat, drink, smoke, breathe, or otherwise come in contact with—known or thought to promote susceptibility to disease. Some programs also teach practices such as the breast self-examination.

Health screening programs are a specific kind of education effort. They provide people with a fairly nonthreatening physical assessment and counseling session in which they can, with a health professional, explore individual cancer risk factors related to diet, smoking, stress, and family history. The major purposes of all primary prevention programs are to help people learn to control their own health habits and seek treatment early. Establishing a climate of trust early on in the relationship with the patient and family can make a significant contribution to the patient's sense of security.

Nurse as teacher

One way hospitalized patients gain a sense of control over their situation is to acquire information about the hospital environment. Knowing who the people are who enter and leave the room, what these people do, what can be expected from each day's events, and basic information about the location of the cafeteria, the schedule of meal deliveries, and other services helps patients adjust and lessens their tension. As an ally in this foreign territory, the nurse educates patients to help them develop effective coping skills in this new situation.

In the diagnostic phase, the nurse develops a plan of care so that the patient has a clear understanding of the tests the physician will order and their sequence. On the basis of the plan, the nurse develops a strategy for teaching the patient the purpose of each test and the preparation and steps of the procedures. Patients usually want to know if diagnostic tests will produce pain or discomfort and when the results will be known. Anticipating patients' needs for information and comfort reassures them that these needs are perfectly normal. It helps them, too, to know that there is an organized plan for their care. Knowing that doctors and nurses have done careful planning helps the patient become assured of their competency and promotes trust.

Including the family in information sharing and education is usually very helpful to all concerned. Teaching the patient and the family together allows more effective participation in care and aids the process of clarifying for each other what was said. Patients should be encouraged to write down questions they wish to ask the physician or nurse, as these questions arise. Often the nurse needs to initiate the questioning because patient or family members may think their questions "dumb" or too trivial to ask of the health-team members.

When the diagnosis of cancer is made and treatment is prescribed, the teaching role of the nurse continues. Patients may undergo surgery that requires a major adjustment in their body image. Radiation therapy, chemotherapy, or special nutritional treatment—all new to the patient—may be prescribed. Throughout treatment, patients encounter a whole new vocabulary, sometimes a new set of care-givers, changes in care needs, and procedures for self-care they and their families must learn. The nurse guides the patient through these new experiences, providing comfort and assurances as part of nursing care.

Coordinator of the health-care team

The best approach to cancer patient care is multidisciplinary: a group of health professionals from different disciplines together planning a comprehensive range of services to combat the disease and assist the patient and family resolve problems that may arise. The composition of the team depends on the resources available in the health-care agency or the community.

The patient's physician directs the course of testing and treatment and communicates these decisions in writing or orally to the patient and family and the rest of the care team. Frequent and complete communication between nurse and physician is essential. The nurse must know what the physician has told the patient and family, and the physician is to be kept informed of the patient's response to treatment and nursing care.

The social worker may assist in placing the patient in a long-term treatment facility if he can't return home following discharge. A social worker can also help the family cope with the financial and emotional stress imposed by the patient's disease. The psychologist or psychiatrist, or both, can provide valuable consultation to the other members of the treatment team, helping them understand the many and varied responses patients and families have to this illness and assisting the staff in planning effective interventions. If indicated, the patient or family as a unit may benefit from some form of problem-centered therapy.

Another central health-care team member is the hospital chaplain or clergyman in the community. Faith in God or a Power greater than oneself can provide a sense of peace and serenity. Patients and their families are likely to ask fundamental questions of life's meaning at the time of cancer diagnosis. A chaplain can be helpful to them in framing their questions and sharing their struggle for answers.

Other professionals may participate in the patient's care either routinely or episodically. The activities of the health-care team require coordination, and the nurse is best situated to perform this function. Because of daily closeness to patient and family, nurses can identify patients' needs for special skills of another professional. In most larger hospitals, the nurse coordinates care given by various professionals in different disciplines who perform specific aspects of patient care. In other settings, the nurse may need to create a team or constellation of professionals and others who can provide the needed services to the patient and family.

Nurse as care provider

The nurse's role as care giver requires correct assessment of patient needs. People entering the hospital for cancer diagnosis or treatment have been living and functioning independently or have returned for care because of an illness crisis or because they have become increasingly dependent on others for assistance. The nurse accommodates to the patients' needs, doing for them what they are unable to do for themselves. The nurse is thus helper to others and shares in very personal and intimate experiences with patients.

— From the patients' perspective, the nurse is a person who is accessible and to whom they can entrust fears and personal concerns during this significant time in their lives. As the patient-nurse relationship develops and continues and as the patients begin treatment, they rely on the nurse for comfort, pain control, or assistance in mastering new self-care procedures, such as colostomy care. In the role of care-giver, the nurse adapts and adjusts care to the patient's changing needs.

The nurse also engages family or friends in the patient's care. Families have reported feeling very useless in providing care and comfort to their loved ones who are hospitalized. Many nurses in cancer care have heard the remark: "At least you can give him medication to relieve the pain." Finding opportunities to engage family members in some care activity, even if it seems insignificant, can be very beneficial to them. For example, rubbing her husband's back can be enormously useful in aiding the wife overcome some of her helpless feelings.

The nursing process

Each person taking on the role of patient enters a different world of relationships, but brings along his or her own set of responses to the world and its realities. "Who is this person?" the nurse asks. "What brings him to the hospital, and what does he need from me?" The patient has a problem, either suspected cancer or need for treatment, and it is the nurse's role to further identify and refine the statement of the patient's problems and develop solutions. The nursing process is a systematic approach to patient care, consisting of assessment, nursing diagnosis, planning, implementation, and evaluation.[3] This process is dynamic and allows adaptation to continuous patient care over time.

ASSESSMENT
This phase of the nursing process begins with the nursing history and ends with a nursing diagnosis. The nurse is expected to identify care problems the patient may have in meeting a wide range of basic human needs and thus must know about normal states and pathophysiology and treatment and nursing care and must understand the medical plan of care. The nurse makes judgments about patients' conditions and

learns to evaluate their perception of their problems. A nursing history is taken as early as possible in the nurse-patient relationship and should be done in an organized manner, following a structured guide. The nurse should be comfortable in interviewing the patient and skillful in directing the interview to an exchange of information on which to base care. In completing a nursing history of cancer patients, the nurse will want to know about family status, significant relationships, whether the patient has had other life crises, what they were, and how he or she coped with them. It's important to learn the patient's own assessment of his or her status, such as the purpose of hospitalization, physical and emotional status, and available resources.

Communications skills and knowledge of disease states and patient responses are basic in obtaining a useful patient history. The history guides the later measurement of body function and physical assessment techniques used to obtain further data. As an outcome of the history and physical assessment, the nurse and patient should have a basic understanding of each other.

In addition to the nursing history and physical assessment, information about the patient may be obtained from the family members, physicians, other health-team members, and records of past hospitalization. Once all information has been obtained, the nurse can analyze it and identify problems or potential problems. A nursing diagnosis is then made, which is a statement of the patient's problems that require nursing intervention.

PLANNING

The next phase of the nursing process results in a plan of care of appropriate nursing responses and interventions. To promote early involvement of patients in their care, as they are able, the nurse includes them in the planning phase as soon as possible. Patients may assist in determining priority problems of most concern to them. For example, a mother of young children who was hospitalized for a diagnostic workup identified the need to have acceptable child-care arrangements before she could concentrate on learning about the diagnostic procedures. The nurse who enables patients to be partners in the development of their plan of care sets a style for nurse-patient interactions in which the patient can gain a sense of control over what happens to him or her, thus enhancing the patient's sense of self-esteem.

Once the patient problems are prioritized, both the patient and the nurse consider possible solutions. Patients may defer to the nurse's clinical expertise, but their solutions must be considered. Together, the nurse and patient try to predict as accurately as possible the outcome of each proposed solution and should select the solution with the most desirable and achievable outcome. This planning is an exercise in goal-setting and includes target dates for implementation and evaluation when feasible. Planning is part of the dynamic nursing process, and, therefore, priorities are evaluated periodically and are reordered as the patient's care needs change.

While many of the prescribed interventions will be performed by the nurse or nurse-designate, some require the involvement of other health professionals. The nurse may make referrals or request that another professional, or perhaps family or friends, assist the patient in resolving one or more problems. As more persons are included in the plan of care, the nurse's role as a care-planning coordinator becomes more important. Designating accountability clearly for different parts of the total plan is necessary when working with members of a health-care team. Coordination and designated accountability prevent gaps in patient-care delivery that can be harmful to patients and families.

Finally, the nursing care plan should be written in a systematic, organized fashion and be available to all health professionals caring for the patient. Although their formats may vary, nursing care plans should include a statement of each of the patient's problems, solutions developed, the designation of nursing interventions, and the desired outcome. The care plan should be reviewed with the physician to assure coordination of the medical and nursing plans of care. A comprehensive statement of the patient's nursing care plan promotes efficient care that engenders trust and confidence in the patient.

IMPLEMENTATION

Implementation of the plan of care is the third phase of the nursing process. This phase presents several challenges to the nurse and is the most visible indication of clinical competence. Nursing care that cancer patients receive requires clinical expertise based on knowledge of normal and disease states and interventions, such as chemotherapy and side-effects of chemotherapeutic agents, pain control and its many nuances, and the signs, symptoms, and treatments of nutritional deficiencies. Advances in cancer nursing occur rapidly, and it is the nurse's responsibility to maintain a high level of competence. It is often difficult to keep abreast of changes in advanced testing and therapies. The ideal facility for comprehensive care of the cancer patient is probably a cancer center with a full range of inpatient and outpatient services, research, and education. But only a few of these exist, and dissemination of new information from these centers takes time. A great majority of patients receive their care in community hospitals and physicians' offices. The professional nurse in these settings must rely on continuing education to be current in knowledge of effective care for cancer patients.

In all care activities, the nurse communicates, through manner and approach, a professional bearing. The more confident, well-prepared, and self-assured the nurse, the safer the patient will feel. Professional judgment and ability are key factors in implementing the nursing care plan. Patients usually describe nurses who convey their confidence and competence as the ones who "know just what to do." Reassuring measures, such as explanations of what is to happen and its purpose, enhance a patient's sense of security and allay fears. The seasoned professional nurses know their own limitations, and call on other resources for consultation. In some instances, another professional may more appropriately implement a part of the plan.

The implementation phase is action-oriented, and assessing, planning, and evaluating occur continuously as care is delivered. For example, the nurse notes the very relaxing effect a backrub has on the patient, and further notes a lessening of the patient's perceived pain. The nurse then prescribes a backrub to relax the patient in preparation for sleep. Thus, implementation is evaluated, leads to new assessments, revisions in planning, and improved care. The nurse records each action and its outcome as a basis for evaluation as time goes on.

EVALUATION

The core questions the nurse asks in evaluating the plan relate to whether the patient's response to the treatment has promoted or hindered progress toward the planned goals and desired outcomes. As coordinator of care and the continuous care giver, the nurse recognizes the outcomes of nursing care and of interventions of other health professionals. The patient, the nurse, other health-team professionals, and family members who are involved in the development of a multidisciplinary plan are evaluators of its effectiveness. The nursing-care plan thus is evaluated singly and also in conjunction with the patient's total plan of care. At the level of the practicing nurse, the evaluation component of the nursing process represents an opportunity for nurses to measure the quality of their own practice. At the level of the health-care team, regularly scheduled conferences for patient evaluation by health-team members represent an opportunity to measure the quality of interdependent care functions.

When involved with cancer patients, nurses are tested professionally and personally. The expectations of patients, families, physicians, and oneself may be at times overwhelming. Nurses caring for cancer patients must be prepared to confront issues that test their attitudes toward their own mortality and vulnerability. To cope with this challenge, nurses must develop a support system. Whether they meet formally in a support group with other cancer nurses and professionals or create a network of support from family, friends or clergy, nurses' personal emotional needs should be addressed in order for them to develop and maintain professional effectiveness. The compelling needs of patients can drain the nurse's physical, emotional, and psychological energy, as can the all-too-frequent experience of patient death. An institution or program that strives to provide competent, humane care to patients and families must also provide a caring environment for nurses.

There is a kind of bonding that takes place when a nurse and patient enter into a care alliance. From the point of view of patients, they experience an advocate whose knowledge enlightens them, and whose reassurance and care comfort them. For the nurse, this care experience reaffirms the rightness of the choice of nursing as a profession.

REFERENCES

1. CANCER FACTS & FIGURES. New York: American Cancer Society, 1980.
2. **Henderson V.** THE NATURE OF NURSING. New York: Macmillan, 1966.
3. **Yura H and Walsh M.** THE NURSING PROCESS, 3rd ed. New York: Appleton-Century-Crofts, 1978.

2
PREVENTION, SCREENING, AND EARLY DETECTION

LINDA DOTSON, RN, BSN

This chapter contains information about risk factors, early detection, and screening methods, and findings and information about cancer prevention and detection. Guides to patient education are presented for selected cancers. All nurses have opportunities to use this information. Nurses in any health-care setting can intervene in the important phases of prevention and early detection of cancer. Just as a nurse is alert to risk factors and signs and symptoms of other diseases such as cardiovascular disease, the nurse also is alert to the risk factors, signs, and symptoms of cancer.

Health-education programs

To use in all of their patient contacts, nurses can draw information from health-education programs about cancer as well as from their knowledge of cancer nursing. Health-education programs are designed to heighten public awareness about cancer and to increase patients' readiness to seek diagnosis and treatment when indicated. Patients may ask nurses to clarify or interpret information learned from health-education programs. Nurses may refer to these programs when teaching patients about cancer.

Health-education programs include a broad scope of activities that pertain to the first phases in the health-illness continuum: prevention, screening, and early detection. National programs for cancer education include television, magazine, and newspaper advertisements designed to make people aware of cancer and the importance of prevention and early detection. Some health-education programs are targeted to communities. Screening programs at health fairs, in conjunction with local public events, or conducted by health agencies specifically for cancer are examples. Programs about cancer presented at meetings of clubs or groups in the community and in schools and industry are also designed to increase people's readiness to act for prevention or early diagnosis. Printed materials provided by the American Cancer Society and other groups are used in these programs and are also distributed in clinics, doctors' offices, and other places where people are likely to pick them up and read them. Nurses, in addition to individual patient teaching, may participate in planning or conducting health-education programs in the community.

Cancer prevention

Nurses should be alert for opportunities to teach patients what is involved in cancer prevention and early detection. The outcome standard for cancer nursing practice in prevention and early detection, as determined by the Oncology Nursing Society and the American Nurses' Association, is that the patient and family possess adequate information about cancer prevention and detection.

PRIMARY PREVENTION
Cancer prevention can be divided into primary and secondary prevention. Primary prevention is taking steps to avoid the disease before it starts. It relates to identifying and dealing with factors that cause or may cause cancer. Many cancers are believed to be associated with physical surroundings, life-style, or personal habits. Their risk factors are identified through observation and research. When risk factors are abated or eliminated, an involved person's potential for developing

cancer is decreased. Some risk factors, such as smoking, can be eliminated. Others, such as age, cannot. Epidemiologic research attempts to identify risk factors and propose possible ways to counteract or eliminate them.

Current information about trends discovered by epidemiologic research and already established facts are used to identify groups of people at high risk for developing cancer. Some studies of the causes of cancer are focused on laboratory research and others on populations known to be at risk. One example of laboratory research is a study of populations with specific types of cancer to locate common factors in their disease through bioassay methods. Another is testing the carcinogenicity of certain chemicals in laboratory animals to determine their potential for causing cancer in humans.

Identification of individuals with high risk for cancer and those with precancerous conditions or lesions known to undergo malignant change is another component of prevention. Women with dysplasia of the cervix, for example, have a 1,600 times greater risk for developing cancer of the cervix than the normal population. Excision of cancer in situ has been observed to prevent invasive carcinoma of the cervix.[1] Individuals with inherited heightened susceptibility to conditions known to be cancer precursors are also identified. Xeroderma pigmentosum, an autosomal recessive disease characterized by exaggerated sensitivity to sunlight, is an example of a condition known to be linked with increased risk of skin cancer early in life. Minimizing exposure to carcinogens and monitoring for incidence of precancerous lesions are means used to counteract or eliminate risks.

SECONDARY PREVENTION

Secondary prevention follows upon cancer detection, specifically when the cancer is discovered with early diagnosis. Secondary prevention is the "diagnosis and removal of cancerous lesions before metastases have developed, and in the case of a premalignant lesion, before it becomes malignant."[2]

Early detection is important for controlling cancer. Treatment is most effective in people younger than age 50 whose cancers were detected early. One of the purposes of cancer health-education programs is to inform people how to recognize suspicious signs and symptoms of cancer in themselves and to seek diagnosis if they occur. Informed patients may thus detect their own cancers early. Cancer may also be detected during a physical examination or during treatment for another health problem. Screening programs are designed specifically to find cancer early. Detection of a localized, curable cancer or precancerous lesion may result from participation in a screening program. Patients with cancer detected in earlier stages live longer after diagnosis and treatment than those with advanced cancers.

A limitation in screening is lack of inexpensive tests that are reliable for early detection. There is some research directed to develop tests that can be used easily, are inexpensive, and are accurate in detection. But at present, screening programs incorporate known information about early signs and symptoms with the tests that are available.

Screening programs are based on the premises that:

- the disease has certain identifiable characteristics;
- there are cost-effective methods and screening tests to detect certain cancers;
- the public must be made aware of these tests and their value in prevention; and
- populations or groups of patients with high potential risk for developing certain types of cancers can be located.

Screening the entire population for cancer could be very costly, but when used appropriately for groups known to have increased probability for developing certain types of cancer, it can be cost-effective and successful in early detection.

Some criteria to be considered in determining the appropriateness of screening tests for early detection are that the tests be:

- available and applicable to many people;
- inexpensive;
- easy to apply and technically simple;
- reproducible;
- of proven value (evidence that early diagnosis for the particular cancer screened in fact increases cure rates);
- accurate in early detection;
- productive of quickly attainable results;
- not painful (tests that are uncomfortable will be avoided); and
- administered by nurses who can also do preventive teaching (physician availability and expense would increase costs).[26]

CANCER PREVENTION AND THE NURSE

Public awareness about cancer is the basis for cancer prevention efforts of all types. Only when misconceptions and fears are dispelled and sufficient, correct information is learned by people, can they make intelligent decisions about what preventive action to take. People should have enough information to recognize that a decision should be made. Even though correct and adequate information about cancer does not necessarily lead to effective prevention, it is a prerequisite for preventive behaviors.

In the remainder of this chapter, information necessary for nurses to correctly assess and teach patients in early phases of cancer care is outlined for the more frequently occurring cancers. This information can enhance your competence in the following areas:

- knowledge of cancer and its natural course;
- knowledge of possible risk factors associated with each of the common sites of cancer;
- ability to take a good history;
- physical assessment skills; and
- knowledge of accessible resources for referral.

Guide to Nursing Care

You can use the information here as a guide in taking a nursing history and in physical assessment while conducting a screening examination for cancer prevention and detection and for patient education. For each of the common cancers, information is given about site, incidence, risk factors, physical findings, detection methods, and prevention, including self-detection methods and recommendations for improved health-care practices.

SKIN (Table 2-1—see page 16)

Nonmelanomatous skin cancer is one of the most common cancers. Each year, there are approximately 400,000 new cases.[6] Because these cancers are directly visible, they are diagnosed earlier, and with adequate treatment there is a 90–95 percent cure rate of basal cell skin cancers. The most common type of skin cancer is basal cell carcinoma; the next is squamous cell carcinoma. Fair-skinned, blue-green and hazel-eyed, reddish-blond-haired individuals seem to be predisposed to developing these types of cancer after chronic, prolonged overexposure to the ultraviolet rays of the sun. Lesions occur most frequently on the exposed surfaces of the body on elderly individuals living in the Sun Belt. There is a much lower occurrence of skin cancer in black people and a very high incidence in individuals with xeroderma pigmentosum.[5]

Melanoma

This skin cancer occurs less frequently than nonmelanomatous skin cancer; there were expected to be approximately 14,800 new cases in 1982.[6] Melanoma is more like a systemic disease because it grows and metastasizes rapidly. Individuals with less pigment in their skin, hair,

TABLE 2-1 SKIN CANCER[3,4,5]

Risk factors	Physical findings
Advanced age; more frequent in males (melanoma can occur in younger age groups but most commonly appears after fifth decade, both sexes). Fair skin. Light eyes (blue, green, hazel). Light hair (blonde, red). Xeroderma pigmentosum. Old burn scars. Radiation exposure (face, acne treatment). Exposure to X-rays, radium, chemical carcinogens—tar, pitch, arsenic. Presence of nevi, especially junctional nevi in the area of constant irritation— waistline, bra line, shoes. Previous skin cancer.	*Basal and squamous cell* cancers may appear as pale, waxlike, pearly nodules; ulcerations or crusty, scaly red outlined patches on lips, scalp, nose, eyelids, cheeks, trunk, hands, arms, legs, and feet.
Environmental: Living in Sun Belt. Chronic overexposure to ultraviolet rays of the sun. Occupations: farmer, sailor, rancher.	*Malignant melanoma:* Pigmented lesions should be given special attention, especially those on legs, trunk, neck, palms, soles, nail beds; nevi subject to irritation, mucous membranes, and genitalia.
Premalignant lesions: Senile keratosis. Leukoplakia. Arsenical keratosis. Nevi subjected to chronic irritation.	Lesions can be flat, raised, brown, black, bluish, red, bluish-red, or combination; irregular border (pigment leaking into surrounding skin, satellite lesions).

and eyes tend to be predisposed to developing melanoma. Those of Northern European descent who burn and freckle when exposed to the sun seem to be at a greater risk. When melanoma occurs in dark-skinned people, it is usually in those areas of less pigmentation, such as the soles of the feet, palms of the hands, and mucous membranes. Sun overexposure and limited pigmentation are risk factors; actual causative factors are still unknown.

Other Skin Lesions
It's important to remember when examining the skin for the common tumors that it is a site for metastasis of other tumors, particularly mel-

Screening & Detection	Patient education
After thorough history, examine entire skin surface with good light source by inspection, palpation; be alert to lesions that have undergone a change in color, diameter, outline, shape, surface, especially flat raised lesions. Ask about itching. Examine regional lymph nodes (melanoma and squamous cell carcinoma). Individuals at high risk should have an eye exam (melanoma). Excision and biopsy of premalignant or suspicious lesions should be done.	High-risk individuals should be cautioned to avoid exposure to the sun. Teach patient to: • inspect skin frequently for changes, using mirror and good light; • use sunscreens with para-amino benzoic acid (PABA); • wear protective clothing (long sleeves and hats); and • avoid sun between hours of 11 and 3, and have patient arrange periodic skin exams with physician or clinic. Give written material on skin cancer and preventive measures.

anoma and cancer of the lung, colon, kidney, and breast. Also, skin lesions can appear with vascular, connective, muscle, and reticuloendothelial cancers. Cancers of adenexal structures, such as sweat gland adenocarcinoma, are rare.

HEAD AND NECK (Table 2-2—see page 20)

Head and neck tumors are grouped together into one category because they tend to have similar etiology and patterns of metastasis. In general, too, diagnostic tests and treatments and rehabilitation of the patient are also similar.

TABLE 2-2 HEAD AND NECK CANCER[4,5,7,8]

Site	Risk factors	Physical findings
Oral cavity (mouth, lip, tongue, buccal mucosa, salivary gland, naso-oropharynx)	Higher incidence in males than females and in ages 60–80. Chewing tobacco and smoking cigarettes, cigars, pipes; excess alcohol intake acts as potentiator of smoking. Repeated trauma from ill-fitting dentures, sharp jagged teeth, and decay. Poor oral hygiene. Overexposure to sunlight (lip). Chronic infections, syphilitic glossitis, stomatitis due to nutritional deficiency, avitaminosis B-6. Genetic predisposition (Chinese ancestry—oropharynx). Premalignant lesions: leukoplakia, erythroplasia.	Most early cancers of this area do not look like cancers. They are often minute ulcers, or areas of slight irritation or thickening. If persistent for more than one month, should be biopsied. In advanced stage, there is elevated fungating mass, flat verrucous tumor, or ulcer in area of thickened tissues. Pain in jaw or teeth, presence of pressure, paresthesia. Bloody nasal discharge. Possible enlarged lymph node. Presence of sore with or without pain. Dysphagia.
Larynx	Cigarette smoking. Polyps on vocal cords.	Persistent hoarseness. Chronic red, sore throat. Growth on vocal cords.
Thyroid	Radiation for benign condition at early age (predominant during the 1940s and 1950s)—for enlarged thymus (infancy), enlarged tonsils, and acne. Affects females more than males. Iodine deficiency and excess.	Generalized swelling in front of neck. Nodules or firm, hard lump. Possible hoarseness. Possible disturbance in thyroid function; signs of hyperthyroidism.

Screening & detection	Patient education
After thorough history, examine oropharynx by inspection and palpation. To inspect tongue, grasp tongue with gauze, pull forward to expose lateral borders while retracting cheek with tongue blade. Glove and palpate for swelling, roughness, induration, and asymmetry. Carefully palpate cheeks, submental and submandibular areas of gums. Use mirror to observe back of mouth and pharynx. Always check neck and cervical lymph nodes. Teach patient normal findings and abnormal findings as examining. Refer to physician for evaluation and possible biopsy of leukoplakia (white patch) and erythroplakia (red patch).	Teach patient warning signs of oral cancers. Develop care plan with patient relative to history, physical exam, and risk factors. Instruct patient to: • do monthly self- exam; • see dentist; • use sunscreen and wear protective clothing; • stop smoking; • decrease alcohol intake; and • maintain good oral hygiene. Give patient written information.
Indirect or direct laryngoscopy by qualified physician.	Give patient information to read. Encourage patient to stop smoking.
After thorough history, examine neck by palpation at rest and while swallowing. Observe swallowing. Cancer centers have established screening clinics for those who were exposed to radiation. Other detection methods: • thyroid scan, • needle aspiration of nodule or lump, and • blood tests to determine abnormal functioning of thyroid.	Provide patient with appropriate information regarding history and personal risk factors. Refer to cancer center for evaluation in thyroid clinic. If patient is high-risk, give written information of both thyroid cancer and signs and symptoms of thyroid pathology.

The American Cancer Society estimates 6 percent of all cancers in males and 2 percent in females are oral cancer, with 27,000 new cases expected in 1982.[6] Oral cancers are those on the lip, tongue, buccal mucosa, floor of mouth, naso-oropharynx, salivary glands, and gums.

Neck tumors are those of the thyroid and the larynx, each with 10,000 cases expected in 1982.[6]

LUNG (Table 2-3—see page 21)

An estimated 129,000 new cases and 111,000 deaths from lung cancer were projected for 1982.[6] This type of cancer is difficult to screen and diagnose early. Consequently, efforts need to be directed toward prevention. Cigarette smoking and respiratory carcinogens, especially asbestos in the work place, are major contributors to lung cancer. Eliminating smoking and taking protective measures against environmental work hazards may reduce incidence and mortality from lung cancer.

Current studies of asymptomatic populations screened for lung cancer by chest roentgenograms and sputum cytology do not show evidence of a notable reduction in mortality from the disease.[5,10]

GASTRIC (Table 2-4—see page 22)

Gastric cancer was expected to account for 24,000 new cases in 1982.[6] For reasons unknown, gastric cancer in the United States is declining. It has been hypothesized that an increase in consumption of wheat cereals that are preserved with antioxidants butylated hydroxytolene (BHT) and butylated hydroxganisole (BHA) is contributory.[5,9] Gastric cancer is difficult to diagnose early.

PROSTATE (Table 2-5—see page 23)

Prostate cancer is the second most common cancer in men. For 1982, 73,000 new cases were projected.[6] Early diagnosis is difficult. Frequently, symptoms bring the patient to seek medical attention. Research is being done to improve the efficiency of blood tumor markers and their significance in early diagnosis.

TESTICULAR (Table 2-6—see page 24)

Testicular cancer is rare, with approximately 5,300 cases expected in 1982.[6] It occurs most frequently in men in upper socioeconomic levels and rarely in blacks or Asians. The average age of occurrence is 32 years. Routine self-examination is probably the best method for early detection.

TABLE 2-3 LUNG CANCER[4,5,8,9]

Risk factors	Physical findings	Screening & detection	Patient education
Heavy cigarette smoking—20 years or more. Exposure to asbestos for those who smoke, risk is eight times that of the nonsmoker who has been exposed, because asbestos acts synergistically with cigarette smoking. Other occupational exposures: auto, chemical, mining occupations—iron ore, nickel, bis (chloromethyl) ether, chromium, uranium, fluorspan, haloether, petroleum. Old scars from lung infections. Smoking and family history of lung cancer. Smoking and history of two or more incidents of pneumonia in one year.	Early lung cancer is often asymptomatic. Auscultation of chest may disclose a unilateral wheeze. Patients often present with persistent productive coughs, hemoptysis, weight loss of 10 lbs in previous six months, repeated bronchitis, pneumonia, lung abscess, chest pain, emphysema, fungal infection, and TB.	Take careful history, including detailed current and past history of smoking habits, respiratory environment of home and work place. Latent period of 20 years between asbestos exposure and occurrence. Screening and early detection methods are limited. PA and lateral chest X-ray. Sputum cytology (value is questionable). CAT scan of lung. Fiberoptic bronchoscopy with biopsy.	*Preventive measures* Provide patient with information on lung cancer and smoking based on personal risk factors. Recommend an annual chest X-ray for those who are at high risk. Review causes and warning symptoms. Provide resource and referral agencies on smoking cessation. Encourage reduced tar intake by changing to lower-tar-content cigarette. Review occupational safety measures.

TABLE 2-4 GASTRIC CANCER[4,5,8,9,11]

Risk factors	Physical findings	Screening & detection	Patient education
Age. Affects male more than female. Blood type group A (20 percent more than those with group 0).	Abdominal tenderness in 20 percent of those examined. Weight loss of 10 pounds or more in previous six months. Black tarry stools in absence of iron supplement. Anorexia. Vomiting blood. All of these could be warning signs of stomach cancer but could also occur with other illnesses. If mass palpated, refer to physician; probably late stage.	Difficult to diagnose early. Thorough history, physical exam. Abdominal palpation on those individuals in high-risk category. Radiologic examination (GI series, CAT scan). Gastroscopy (fiberoptic). Endoscopy. Biopsy. Exfoliative cytology. Abnormal CBC may indicate other conditions. Hemacult slide (fecal) may indicate other conditions.	Should be focused on high-risk individual. Give patient written information on risk factors and warning signs. Dietary counseling: • reduce amount of smoked fish and meat and nitrate additives; • increase amount of vitamin C vegetables; and • reduce alcohol intake. Recommend annual physical examination for people 40 years and older (every three years for those aged 20–39).
History of gastric ulcer, atrophic gastric mucosa, pernicious anemia, prior gastric resection for ulcer disease.			
Polyps in stomach (premalignant condition).			
Certain dietary associations—smoked fish, meat, and common use of foods with nitrate additives.			
Lower socioeconomic level.			
Affects more nonwhites, than whites.			
Higher index of suspicion in residents of Chile, Japan, Iceland, and Poland.			

TABLE 2-5 PROSTATE CANCER[4,5,12,13]

Risk factors	Physical findings	Screening & detection	Patient education
Age: 60–70 years. Higher incidence in blacks. Family history of prostate cancer. Higher incidence in those living in urban areas, which suggests possible environmental causes. History of benign disease and/or prostatitis does not necessarily increase risks.	Unless you're experienced, in digital rectal examination, a nurse specialist or physician should examine. Explain procedure to patient. Note irregularities on right lateral position and left lateral rectal wall. Turn hand so the rectal surface can be examined with finger. Note the lateral lobes and median sulcus. Describe size, shape, consistency; hard irregular nodule and asymmetry may indicate a tumor.	Take complete history, including history of hypertrophy. Repeated infections. VD. Difficulty with urination. Obstruction (starting stream, dribbling, post-micturition pain, or other symptoms). Digital rectal exam is most accurate and cost-effective mass screening method. Tests that may indicate later stages of cancer are: • acid phosphatase enzyme, • acid phosphatase (RIA), • acid phosphatase (CIEP), • urine cytology before and after massage, • urine cytology—aspiration, • prostatic secretion cytology after massage, and • prostatic biopsy.	Discuss with patient findings and risk factors. Recommend annual digital rectal exam for men over age 40. Patient should seek medical attention if symptoms occur.

TABLE 2-6 TESTICULAR CANCER[5,13,14]

Risk factors	Physical findings	Screening & detection	Patient education
Age: 20–40 years. History of undescended testes (cryptorchidism) (1 in 80 inguinal and 1 in 20 abdominal testes will become malignant). Atrophic testes, hernia-genitourinary tract anomalies. Trauma. Orchitis (mumps). Genetic factors. Endocrine abnormalities. Previous cancer of the testes. Possible DES-exposed mother.	If you are inexperienced in bimanual exam of scrotal contents, refer to physician or nurse specialist. Note size and if swollen. Palpate each testis; note size, consistency, shape, and tenderness. Note any nodules. If swelling is present, evaluate by transillumination. In dark, shine penlight from behind scrotum; if normal, will be red glow. Any nodule must be evaluated further. Palpate inguinal lymph nodes.	Take complete history; ask specific questions about previous trauma or mumps, heaviness, swelling, or pain in testes. Physical examination—bimanual palpation of scrotum. Biopsy. Surgery for cryptorchidism before age six may reduce risk. Some men with testicular cancer have elevated serum HCG, AFP, and LH levels possibly up to six months prior to clinical manifestation of the tumor; however, negative values do not exclude tumor at this point, so they are not valuable for early screening and detection.	Patient should learn self-exam and understand rationale for practicing routine monthly examination and report any changes. Counseling and plan for education will be based on physical exam, history, and personal risk factors.

TABLE 2-7 BLADDER CANCER[4,5,9,15]

Risk factors	Physical findings	Screening & detection	Patient education
Age: 50–70 years. Affects males more than females (3:1). Occupational exposure to chemical carcinogens: beta and alpha naphthylamine, benzidine, 4 aminodiphenyl and 4 nitro diphenyl, auramine, chlornaphazine. Smoking. Hydroxylkynurenine and 3 hydroxyanthralinic acid are thought to promote bladder cancer. Abnormal tryptophane metabolism found in some patients with recurrent bladder tumors. Bilharziasis caused by viruses (RNA). Schistosomiasis. Constant cystitis with inflammation by calculus. Bladder diverticulum. Family history. Blood type group A. Controversial: excessive use of coffee and drinks with artificial sweeteners.	Patient may present with urinary tract symptoms: intermittent gross hematuria (painless), frequency, urgency, dysuria. Weight loss. Abdominal mass. Enlarged regional lymph nodes.	Take thorough history, including occupational and personal factors; physical exam: abdominal palpation, bimanual exam in the female, digital rectal exam in male; examine regional lymph nodes. Complete urinalysis. If findings positive, further testing might include cystoscopy, urine cytology. Biopsy, cytologic smear.	Prevention plan for patient is based on history, physical findings, and risk factors. Review occupational exposure risks: dye and paint manufacture, leather, food, cable, asphalt, coal, pitch, and tar industries. Review warning signs and symptoms; patient should seek medical attention immediately if symptoms occur. Review rationale for smoking cessation and reduction of intake of excessive amounts of coffee and drinks with saccharin. Industrial, public health, and community nurses are in the position to develop mass education and screening programs to reduce the incidence of bladder cancer.

TABLE 2-8 GYNECOLOGICAL CANCER[5,8,16–19]

Site	Risk factors	Physical findings
Cervix	Early coitus. Multiple sexual partners. Chronic trichomonas. Vaginal infections. Low socioeconomic status. STD including syphilis and herpes genitalia. Uncircumcised partner.	You may see erosion on cervix.
Vagina	DES-exposed in utero. Age: 14 years or older.	Red focal areas on vagina. Indurated, firm, cystic areas in vagina, cervix. Note discharge and presence of leukoplakia and kraurosis.
Endometrium	Age: over 40. History of: obesity, hypertension, diabetes. Infertility. Irregular menses. Failure to ovulate. Endometrial hyperplasia. History of receiving estrogens for menopausal symptoms. Family history of endometrial cancer.	Enlarged boggy uterus.

Screening & detection	Patient education
Take complete history with accurate details of menstrual, obstetric, gynecologic, and sexual activity. Get history of infections, sexually transmitted diseases, contraception methods, estrogen therapy, and previous Pap results. Pelvic exam should be done by experienced examiner.	Care plan should be designed according to individual's risk factors, history, and physical findings. Recommend physical exam and Pap smears based on risk factors. The American Cancer Society recommends Pap tests should be done every three years, after two consecutive Pap tests done a year apart with negative results for women 20–40 years of age, or younger if sexually active, and annually for women over 40. The same recommendations apply for pelvic exams. These recommendations are controversial. In general, teaching should be directed toward getting the information on screening to the high-risk population in order to change or improve their health-care practices.
Inspect vulvovaginal area.	
Inspect cervix and take Pap smears from endocervical canal, cervix, and vaginal pool. Do bimanual examination of uterus and adnexa: note size, shape, consistency, tenderness, and mobility. Palpate ovaries and rectovaginal area. If there are abnormal findings, further tests may include: • Schiller's test • colposcopy-biopsy and • endometrial aspiration, biopsy, curettage.	Patients with known risk factors should have a routine physical examination as indicated. In addition, the American Cancer Society recommends that those women at menopause with risk factors should have an endometrial tissue sample taken.

Continued on next page.

TABLE 2-8 continued

Site	Risk factors	Physical findings
Ovary	Age: 50–70 (post-menopausal). Upper socioeconomic status. History of reduced fertility or infertility. History of breast cancer. Family history of breast, ovarian, colon cancer.	Abdominal distention, lower abdominal pain. Mass, usually bilateral, with fixed, irregular shape. Adnexal thickening (especially in postmenopausal and nulliparous women). On examination, cul-de-sac may feel like "handful of knuckles."

BLADDER (Table 2-7—see page 25)

Bladder cancer accounts for about 37,000 cases of cancer per year.[6] Available data suggest that bladder cancer has multiple etiologies.[4] Many people diagnosed with bladder cancer live in industrialized areas, suggesting exposure to certain chemical carcinogens. A few carcinogens have been shown to cause bladder cancer, and measures have been taken against them, but there is a latent period after exposure, with some bladder tumors developing several years later.[5]

GYNECOLOGICAL CANCER (Table 2-8—see page 26)

The most common gynecologic cancers are those of the cervix, uterus, corpus uteri, and ovary. The American Cancer Society estimated 16,000 cases of invasive carcinoma of the cervix, 39,000 cases of endometrial cancer, and 18,000 cases of ovarian cancer would be diagnosed in 1982.[6] Less common lesions are found in the vulva and vagina, with 4,400 cases estimated for 1982.

Although the evidence is not conclusive, it strongly indicates that the early detection of cervical cancer with a Pap test reduces mortality from the disease, and in fact actually prevents invasive cervical cancer by detecting its precursors, severe dysplasia and carcinoma in situ.[8] For those women at high risk for developing endometrial cancer, an aspiration cytology test of a tissue sample is available for possible discovery of pre-clinical disease. A complete gynecologic examination is basic to early detection of all gynecologic malignancies. Careful in-

Screening & detection	Patient education
Pap, cul-de-sac tap, (culdocentesis), ultrasonography, laparoscopy, biopsy. Current research shows potential for serologic test for earlier detection.	

spection and bimanual pelvic exam may detect vulvovaginal lesions and ovarian masses, which are malignancies that are sometimes difficult to detect early.

BREAST (Table 2-9—see page 30)

Breast cancer affects one out of 11 women in the United States; 112,000 women and 900 men were expected to be diagnosed in 1982 as having breast cancer.[6] Breast cancer is the most common cancer in women and the No. 1 cancer killer in women of any age. Screening for breast cancer appears to offer promise of reduced mortality. It's known that when breast cancer is clinically localized before nodal involvement, the five-year survival rate is 85 percent. The survival rate decreases with a nodal involvement.[20,22] Ninety percent of breast tumors are discovered by the patient. Until breast cancer can be prevented, the greatest hope for control is early detection. Emphasis must be placed on breast self-exam.

COLON AND RECTAL CANCER (Table 2-10—see page 32)

Colon and rectal cancers are the second most frequently occurring cancer and are the largest group of gastrointestinal cancers. Both sexes are affected, and survival depends on the stage of the disease at the time of diagnosis. Estimated occurrences for 1982 were 83,000 new cases of colon and 38,000 new cases of rectal cancer.[6]

TABLE 2-9 BREAST CANCER[4,5,9,15,19–22]

Risk factors	Physical findings
Female (1:11), rare in males. Age: over 40. Family history of breast cancer, especially mother, sister, or aunt. Personal history of breast cancer. Benign breast disease: chronic cystic mastitis, intraductal papilloma, fibrocystic disease. Nulliparous. First pregnancy after the age of 30. Early menarche. Late menopause. Endometrial cancer. Immunodeficiency. Obesity, diabetes, hypertension. Use of exogenous estrogens and hypertensive agents (questionable). Adverse hormonal milieu. Possibly chronic psychological stress. *Environmental:* Cold climate. Western hemisphere. White race. Upper socioeconomic status. Excessive ionizing radiation. Viruses. High fat diet, especially milk fat.	Often noted by patient in breast self-exam. Changes noted on inspection: • size, shape, symmetry, and direction of nipple pointing (inversion) when inspecting breasts in front of a mirror (sitting or standing) with arms raised above head and pectoral muscles contracted and in changing arm positions; • dimpling, puckering, skin changes, edema, red patches, orange texture. Change noted on palpation: • in supine position, discharge from breast when pressing or squeezing nipple; • detection of nodules when palpating breast using circular, rotating motion—cancer or tumors tend to be hard, irregular in shape, and fixed often in upper outer quadrant.

Screening & detection	Patient education
Breast self-exam. Breast exam by nurse examiner or physician. Mammography. Thermography. Graphic stress test. Research is under way to determine the value of biochemical screening, specifically androgen and estrogen ratios and levels in serum and urine.	Breast self-exam (BSE) is the most important method in early detection. Share information with patient about breast cancer, her own personal risk factors in manner that enhances an understanding of her body and possible susceptibility, but does not provoke excessive anxiety precluding willingness to do BSE. Review risk factors and anatomy with patient. Review BSE with films, posters. Have patient demonstrate BSE. Emphasize the importance of regular, monthly BSE: premenopausal—on the day menses cease; postmenopausal or patients who have had a hysterectomy—on the first of each month. If changes are noted, patient should see physician. The American Cancer Society recommends a baseline mammogram for patients age 35–40, especially if symptomatic or at risk. Patients over 50 should have an annual mammogram. Another recommendation is that all women over 20 years do monthly BSE; women 20–40 should have exam by physicians every three years; and women over 40 should have annual examinations by physician. Review nutrition with patient, especially with regard to dairy product fats and red meat intake.

TABLE 2-10 RECTAL CANCER[4,8,9,19,23–25]

Risk factors	Physical findings	Screening & detection	Patient education
Age: over 40 years. Familial colonic polyposis, Gardner syndrome (polyps), adenomatous polyps (premalignant). Family history of colon cancer. History of colitis for 10 years. Diets high in fat and meat, low in fiber. Possible history of cholecystectomy. Higher incidence in industrial countries.	Abdominal palpation and digital rectal exam may find mass. Physician may discover lesion in colorectal areas during proctosigmoidoscopy. Positive hemocult slide test indicates necessity of further workup.	During history, ask about changes in bowel habits and in size or caliber of stool, constipation, diarrhea, abdominal pain, rectal bleeding, loss of appetite, weight loss, malaise. Physical exam includes abdominal palpation, digital rectal exam. Fecal occult blood test. Complete blood count. Proctosigmoidoscopy and colonoscopy may be indicated to examine colorectal areas. Early—colon X-ray; barium enema may be indicated. CEA is not specific but sometimes elevated in advanced disease. Biopsy.	Preventive teaching includes a review and discussion of anatomy, warning signs, and symptoms. The American Cancer Society recommends all persons over 40 should have a digital rectal exam annually. Stool for guiac test should be done annually for those over 50. Sigmoidoscopy should be performed every three to five years after two initial negative sigmoidoscopies one year apart. High-risk individuals should be examined more frequently or as determined by their physician.

Summary

Information presented in this chapter includes an overview of risk factors, prevention, screening, and detection methods for selectd common cancer sites. Because cancer research is always advancing, you should maintain a source of current information about new discoveries in cancer care. There is always progress in the detection of potential health hazards—new information about the effects of environmental factors in the occurrence of cancer and in testing of new products such as chemicals before their widespread use. There is progress, too, in the development of preventive agents such as retinoids, selenium compounds, and antioxidants. You should be aware of these significant efforts. The important focus of nursing care, however, is the patient. Educating the patient about personal risks, warning signals, the importance of physical examination, and self-detection methods is prominent in the nurse's role in patient care.

REFERENCES

1. **DeVita VT, Hellman S, and Rosenberg SA.** CANCER—PRINCIPLES AND PRACTICES OF ONCOLOGY. Philadelphia: Lippincott, 1982.

2. **Miller DG.** Principles of early detection of cancer, CANCER 47:142, 1981.

3. **Gumport SL, Harris MN, Roses DF, et al.** The diagnosis and management of common skin cancers, CA 31:79, 1981.

4. **Khandekar JD and Lawrence GA.** FUNDAMENTALS IN CANCER MANAGEMENT. Niles, I11: MEL, 1982.

5. **Stromberg MF.** Nursing's contribution: 40 case findings and the early detection of cancer. In CANCER NURSING, Marino LB (ed). St Louis, Mo: Mosby, 1981.

6. CANCER FACTS & FIGURES. New York: American Cancer Society, 1981.

7. THE CHALLENGE OF ORAL CANCER. New York: American Cancer Society, 1975.

8. CANCER-RELATED HEALTH CHECK-UP; 1980 GUIDELINES. New York: American Cancer Society, 1980.

9. **Doll R and Peto R.** THE CAUSE OF CANCER. New York: Oxford University Press, 1981.

10. **National Institutes of Health.** Treating diabetic retinopathy: Guideline for lung cancer screening. JAMA 241:1581, 1979.

11. CANSCREEN RISK FACTOR MANUAL. Philadelphia: Institute for Cancer Research, 1975.

12. **Guinan P, Gilham N, Nagubadi SR, et al.** What is the best test to detect prostate cancer? CA 31:141, 1981.

13. **Bates B.** A GUIDE TO PHYSICAL EXAMINATION, 2nd ed. Philadelphia: Lippincott, 1979.

14. **Maher ML.** Screening and early detection. Unpublished.

15. **Schottenfeld D and Hass J.** CARCINOGENS IN THE WORK PLACE. New York: American Cancer Society, 1977.

16. **Barber H.** OVARIAN CANCER. New York: American Cancer Society, 1979.

17. **Gusberg SB.** AN APPROACH TO THE CONTROL OF CARCINOMA OF THE ENDOMETRIUM. New York: American Cancer Society, 1980.

18. **Nelson JH, Averette HE, and Richart RM.** DETECTION, DIAGNOSTIC EVALUATION, AND TREATMENT OF DYSPLASIA CARCINOMA IN SITU AND EARLY INVASIVE CERVICAL CARCINOMA. New York: American Cancer Society, 1979.

19. **O'Donnell W, Day E, and Venet L.** EARLY DETECTION AND DIAGNOSIS OF CANCER. St Louis: Mosby, 1962.

20. **Anthony C.** Risk factors associated with breast cancer. NURSE PRAC 3(4):31, July/August 1978.

21. BREAST CANCER DIGEST: A GUIDE TO MEDICAL CARE, EMOTIONAL SUPPORT, EDUCATION PROGRAMS, AND RESOURCES. Washington: National Institutes of Health, 1979.

22. **Marchant DJ.** Breast diseases, CLIN OBSTET GYNECOL 25:387, 1982.

23. **Overholt BF.** Colonoscopy and colon cancer: Current clinical practice. CA 32:180, 1982.

24. **Sherman CD.** CLINICAL CONCEPTS IN CANCER MANAGEMENT. New York: McGraw-Hill, 1976.

25. **Winawer SJ, Fleisher M, Baldwin M.** Current status of occult blood testing in screening for colorectal cancer. CA 32:100, 1982.

26. **Sato P.** The detection of cancer. In DYNAMICS OF ONCOLOGY NURSING, Burkhalter PK and Donley D (eds). New York: McGraw-Hill, 1977.

3
DIAGNOSIS

MICHELLE A. McCLANAHAN, RN, BS
MARY E. MIELNICKI, RN, BSN

Patients enter the diagnostic workup phase soon after they realize they have a problem—or can no longer deny it—and seek medical attention. Patients usually enter the health-care system through referral from a screening program, their physicians, or nurse specialists. During the diagnostic workup, your work with the patient is a combination of emotional support and patient education with physical care. Diagnosis to the potential oncology patient means undergoing a series of blood tests, X-rays, procedures, biopsies and relating to many different care givers, often in an unfamiliar environment.

History and physical examination

The nurse is often one of the first professionals patients and their families meet when entering the hospital system. This initial meeting is the beginning of the nurse-patient relationship, which can be an important source of stability for the patient and family throughout the hospital stay.

Nursing assessment begins at this first meeting. In assessment, the nurse systematically acquires data about the patient and family by asking pertinent questions, making observations, listening and examining. A nursing history is an assessment tool that helps the nurse obtain data about physiologic and psychosocial status. Many standard forms are used to structure the interview questions for getting a patient's history. Figure 3-1 is a sample of such a form. You may obtain the history from the patient, the family, or both. If the patient is accompanied by family members, you can take part of the history with the family present. Observing the interaction among them can give you insight into the relationships and the needs of patient and family. During the interview, observe the patient for signs of physical function, such as breathing patterns, edema, or other visible signs that provide clues to what questions should be emphasized.

There are 10 categories of essential information. They are given here with questions and the rationale for obtaining this information.

Reason for admission
Have the patient describe to you why he or she has come to the hospital. Although you know the admitting diagnosis from the physician, it's important to learn the patient's perceptions of the reasons.

Interview questions. What is your chief complaint? How did you recognize the problem? Have you experienced pain or observed a lump or swelling? How long have you had the symptoms? Have you undergone a diagnostic workup as an outpatient to determine the cause of the symptom?

Expectations of hospitalization
The nurse must remember that patients have their own expectations for hospitalization, developed by previous hospitalizations, from family and friends, and by the media, as well as through information from the physician.

Interview questions. What information has the patient received from the physician? Has the physician told the patient about the possible diagnosis—a tumor, clot, infectious process—and about the diagnostic tests, such as X-rays, blood tests, or other procedures that would be ordered?

Understanding of cancer
If patients are in the hospital to rule out cancer, or if they manifest fear that cancer will be found, explore their understanding of cancer. Because of the widespread attention given to cancer in magazines,

newspapers, and television, a patient may be either well-informed or confused about what cancer is and its prognosis.

Interview questions. Does the patient have a friend or a family member with cancer? Known someone who died of cancer? What is his or her greatest fear about cancer? Does the patient view cancer as a fatal disease? Does the patient think he or she has cancer?

Social background

Through this part of the interview, you get to know the patient's social data. This part of the interview deals with the kind of information that can lead the patient to feel he or she can trust you. You will find the information useful in helping the patient during the diagnostic period and, if indicated by the diagnosis, in later patient decisions about selection of treatment, acceptance of diagnosis, and coping with responses of family, friends, employers, and others.

Interview questions. Is the patient single, married, widowed or divorced, separated? Does he or she have children or other dependents? Who provides the patient with emotional support? Ask the patient: How do you deal with stress? What is your work or career? What are your major interests? The name and phone number of the responsible family member or friend should be recorded.

Past medical history

The patient's past medical history and record of previous hospitalizations are used in planning nursing care for the current admission. The previous medical history is taken by means of interview questions regarding each body system in sequence, including the respiratory, cardiovascular, central nervous, endocrine, genitourinary, gastrointestinal, and sensory systems. Specific questions such as, "Have you ever had a breathing problem?" or "Have you ever had asthma, bronchitis, pneumonia, recurrent colds?" are asked for each system. The patient may be nervous and fail to give accurate information if they feel they are being drilled relentlessly. If you ask the questions in different forms and try to be less repetitious, you may get more accurate information.

In addition to asking questions about signs and symptoms and previous or current illnesses, ask general questions about previous hospitalizations and treatment. Find out whether the patient has previously been hospitalized, had surgery, or had some other form of treatment. Note medications taken previously or currently being taken as well as any drug reactions or allergies.

Interview questions. A list of questions to ask in taking the past medical history is too long to provide here. Texts on assessment can supply you with guidelines for questions you need to ask concerning the body systems. In addition to this information, you should also as-

38

FIGURE 3-1 ADMITTING PATIENT PROFILE FOR NURSING and NURSING DISCHARGE SUMMARY

PATIENT'S NAME				AGE	
OCCUPATION		RELIGION			
ADMITTED TO ROOM	BY (SIGNATURE)	METHOD OF ARRIVAL		DATE	TIME
TEMP.	PULSE ☐REG. ☐IRREG.	RESP.	BP	HEIGHT ☐ACTUAL ☐EST.	WEIGHT ☐ACTUAL ☐EST.
DOCTOR					

1. REASON FOR ADMISSION

2. SIGNS & SYMPTOMS & DURATION

3. EXPECTED LENGTH OF HOSPITALIZATION

4. EXPECTATIONS OF HOSPITALIZZATION

5. PLANS FOR DISCHARGE

6. PRE-EXISTING CONDITIONS:

   ALLERGIES (FOOD & DRUG)

   RESPIRATORY

   CARDIOVASCULAR

   CENTRAL NERVOUS SYSTEM

   ENDOCRINE

GENITOURINARY

GASTROINTESTINAL

DIETARY LIMITATIONS

PHYSICAL DISABILITIES

MECHANICAL DEVICES: ☐ CRUTCHES ☐ CANE ☐ WALKER ☐ PROSTHESIS ☐ DENTURES: ___ FULL ___ PARTIAL

ACTIVITY LIMITATIONS

SENSORY DEFICITS: ☐ GLASSES ☐ CONTACTS ☐ HEARING AID: R   L

EMOTIONAL/PSYCHIATRIC

LEVEL OF CONSCIOUSNESS

MEDICATIONS

SKIN INTEGRITY

7. SLEEP PATTERNS

8. HOW IS HOSPITALIZATION   FAMILY? _____
   AFFECTING THE PATIENT'S   JOB? _____

NURSE'S INITIAL
ASSESSMENT OF
THE PATIENT

ORIENTATION
TO THE UNIT: ☐ BED CONTROLS   ☐ CALLBELL   ☐ PHONE   ☐ DISPOSITION OF VALUABLES

COMMENTS

certain the patient's preferences and habits for daily activities such as hygiene, exercise, diet, and the like. Also, you should refer to the previous records of patients who are being admitted for rehospitalization. Use this information to provide consistency in care regarding diet, activity, treatment, or other nursing care measures from one hospitalization to the next.

Medications
You should ask the patient what medications he or she is taking and compare the patient's response with the physician's record of the patient's medication. The patient may be taking the medications incorrectly or could be medicating himself. Patients' perception of why they are taking a medication is important for assessing their understanding of the medication as well as their need for instruction. In addition, ask all patients if they have any allergic reactions—rash or a respiratory problem—to any medication. If so, ask them to describe the reaction experience.

Interview questions. What medications (pills) are you taking? How many and how often for each medication? Why are you taking the medications? Do you take sleeping pills?

Dietary limitations
The nurse should find out the patient's normal dietary routine; any special likes or dislikes should be recorded for later reference in planning intervention for anorexia from treatment such as chemotherapy or radiation.

Interview questions. Are you on a special diet? What types of foods are included or restricted in the diet? Is it a diabetic or sugar-restricted diet? Are you a vegetarian? What food do you prefer? How frequently do you eat—three meals a day, six meals? Do you have an evening snack before bed?

Special needs
Planning nursing care involves knowing the patient's habits, impairments, preferences, and perceived needs for activities of daily living and communication. Assistive devices the patient requires for ambulation, vision, hearing, eating, or other functions are noted and incorporated into the nursing care plan. The patient may have a prosthesis, require a cane or walker, or may need assistance in ambulation. Help the patient obtain the needed devices if he or she did not bring them to the hospital. Note the patient's use of eyeglasses or contacts, dentures, or hearing aids, and accommodate care measures to the patient's needs for safety, communication, and adaptation to the hospital environment as necessary.

Interview questions. Find out how the patient ambulates. Do you use a walker or a cane or will you need assistance? Do you have a hearing problem? Do you have visual problems? Do you use glasses or contacts? Do you wear dentures?

Emotional needs

Cancer is a difficult disease process to cope with, mainly because of its uncertain prognosis. Definite answers about cures and remission periods can't be given. Therefore, the patient is under great stress, and understanding the patient's previous ways of coping with problems can help you to assist him or her in dealing with hospitalization and diagnosis, and depending on diagnostic outcome, with treatment and chronicity.

Interview questions. Find out what the patient thinks: What are your coping mechanisms? Do you use tranquilizers or alcohol? How much? How often? What do you do when you are angry, depressed? Have you ever seen a psychiatrist? If so, why? Have you ever belonged to a support group? If so, why? Was it helpful? It should be noted that the patient may not respond to these questions and should not be forced to.

When a patient is in pain or under stress, this history can be obtained in sections, to allow time to rest. Many of the questions about coping and views on cancer can be asked during nurse-patient contacts as the patient begins to develop trust in the nurse.

Diagnostic Tests

As part of the initial diagnostic workup, routine blood tests, X-rays, and specimen examinations are usually ordered to assess the patient's health status. These routine tests are not specific for cancer, but the results can indicate the presence of an abnormal condition, such as infection, bleeding, or other pathologic processes associated with cancer, pre-existing conditions, or new pathology that is not cancer. The tests are not described here because they are used in any diagnostic workup. Two blood tests, however—a leukocyte count and the CEA—can strongly indicate the presence of cancer, and if positive, are used with other findings to confirm the diagnosis of cancer. An elevated leukocyte count or an abnormal excess of neutrophils, which are immature leukocytes, along with a predominant type of white cell indicates leukemia. Carcinoembryonic antigen (CEA), discovered in an immunologic study, is a tumor-associated antigen which, when found along with significant results of other tests, indicates Hodgkin's disease.

NURSING CARE DURING DIAGNOSTIC TESTING

Most diagnostic tests are relatively painless and do not cause much lasting discomfort, but they further confirm to the patient that there is reason to be concerned about the diagnosis of cancer. This concern is relieved only when the diagnosis is ruled out. Each test that the patient has, each new person the patient meets, can increase the feeling that he or she is losing control. You can help patients keep control over this unknown environment and also begin a trusting relationship with them by:

- informing them of all tests they will have, even blood draws;
- explaining why the test has been ordered;
- informing them about the location of each testing place; and
- if it is known beforehand, informing them about the time schedule for the tests.

FURTHER DIAGNOSTIC PROCEDURES

After the initial history, physical, and routine tests are completed, further diagnostic procedures are almost always ordered. Many of these procedures require the patient's written permission. Each institution has protocols for obtaining the patient's signed permission. An essential element in these protocols is that before signing, the patient and family must be informed. They need to know:

- what the test involves;
- why the patient needs the test for diagnosis;
- what the risk factors are; and
- whether there are any other options.

In most health-care agencies, the physician who will perform the test explains the procedure and obtains the permission. Your role is to support the patient through the decision process and, if the patient consents, through the testing procedures. Special preparation, such as a special diet, cathartic, or a sedative, is required preparation for many diagnostic procedures. Before preparing the patient, you must assess his or her condition and any expected effects the preparatory requirements may have. Your assessment should include these considerations:

1. What is the patient's basic physical state? Note the presence of dehydration, pain, ability to stand upright, ability to lie flat for at least an hour.
2. What effects does this particular preparation usually have? What is it likely to cause in this patient? Will it cause diarrhea, aggravated bleeding, or increased pain?
3. Is the patient allergic to any of the medications ordered?

4. If the patient's condition is unstable, but the test is essential, should the nurse or physician accompany the patient? What accommodations can be made to ensure the patient's comfort and safety?
5. Does the patient need an IV to treat dehydration? Will medication be needed during the test or to treat side effects afterward?
6. Should the patient have pain medication before the test to promote comfort?

The results of diagnostic tests are evaluated by the physician, and often also by the oncology team, to determine whether the patient has an abnormal condition. Diagnostic tests can be used to rule out the presence of a mass or of particular types of tumors or to locate an abnormal mass. But even after the patient has undergone a battery of tests, a positive diagnosis may still be dependent on surgical procedures. In the following section, the more frequently used diagnostic tests are described along with what these tests imply with regard to nursing care. Procedures in use at Evanston Hospital are presented here as guides, but aspects of diagnostic procedures vary in different health-care agencies.

INTRAVENOUS PYELOGRAM (IVP)

Description: An X-ray examination in which a radiopaque, iodine-containing material administered intravenously is used to demonstrate abnormalities, such as tumors, calculi, strictures, or organ displacement of the kidneys, ureters, and bladder.

Preparation:
1. Iodine allergies (seafood) or allergic reactions to previous iodine tests should be reported to the physician and radiology department.
2. Preparation is ordered by the physician and usually includes, for example, urine specific gravity.
3. Diarrhea, rectal bleeding, or emesis may require an alternate preparation. Consult physician.
4. Physician should be consulted concerning diet and insulin for diabetic patients.
5. Should be done pror to or three days after barium studies.

Patient teaching: 1. Contrast dye is administered slowly, over a 10- to 15-minute period, into a prominent arm vein.
2. Films are taken at intervals with the patient in various positions on the examining table.
3. Examination takes one to four hours.

Implementation: Patient is sent to radiology via wheelchair if ambulatory; otherwise, send by cart.

Evaluation: 1. Allergic reactions should be considered if the patient is allergic to iodine-containing materials. Report to the physician any nausea, vomiting, respiratory distress, flushing, or urticaria.
2. Inspect injection site for signs of infiltration, such as redness, swelling, pain, or a burning sensation. Apply ice to the infiltrated site and notify physician.
3. Hypotension may occur in some patients.
4. To evaluate elimination of the dye, take specific gravity of patient's urine after each voiding until it returns to pretest level.
5. Patient resumes his diet unless otherwise ordered.
6. Encourage fluids unless contraindicated.
7. Repeat test is ordered if visualization was hindered by previous barium studies.
8. Test is interpreted by the radiologist.

UPPER GASTROINTESTINAL SERIES (UGI)

Description: An X-ray examination in which oral administration of barium sulfate and air-producing crystals is used to demonstrate abnormalities, such as stenosis, dilation, motility, growths, ulcers, or organ displacement of the esophagus and stomach. The small intestine is also studied if a "small bowel follow-through" is ordered.

Preparation: 1. Diet is not restricted on the day before the examination.

2. Patients who have had a barium enema within three days may need to clear it with a suds enema the evening before or on the morning of the examination.Test may have to be delayed until three days after a barium enema.
3. Individualized orders are necessary if patient has severe diarrhea or rectal bleeding. Patients who also have emesis may require special consideration.
4. Physician should be consulted concerning diet and insulin for diabetic patients.

Patient teaching:
1. Patient swallows the barium, and X-rays are taken periodically as the barium moves down the gastrointestinal tract.
2. Films are taken at intervals with the patient in various positions on the table.
3. Physician may occasionally press on the patient's abdomen during the test.
4. Examination takes two to three hours.

Implementation: Patient is sent to radiology via wheelchair if ambulatory; otherwise, send by cart.

Evaluation:
1. Oral administration of 4 cc of mineral oil will aid evacuation of the barium from the gastrointestinal tract.
2. Physician should be notified if barium is not eliminated.
3. Repeat test is ordered if visualization was hindered by previous barium studies.
4. Test is interpreted by radiologist.

BARIUM ENEMA WITH LOWER GI X-RAY

Description: An X-ray examination in which a barium sulfate enema is used to demonstrate abnormalities of the large intestine, such as stenosis, dilation, or growths.

Preparation:
1. Diet is usually adjusted the day before as ordered by physician.

2. A cathartic the night before is ordered by physician.
3. NPO after midnight.
4. Diarrhea, rectal bleeding, or emesis may require an alternate preparation; the physician should be consulted.
5. Physician should be consulted concerning diet and insulin for diabetic patients.

Patient teaching:
1. Barium is inserted per enema into large intestine.
2. Radiologist periodically stops the flow and takes pictures.
3. Films are taken at intervals with patient in various positions on the table.
4. Examination takes 15 minutes to one hour.

Implementation: Patient is sent to radiology via wheelchair if ambulatory; otherwise, send by cart.

Evaluation:
1. Stool is observed post-test to be sure that barium is eliminated. Notify physician if it was not passed.
2. Milk of magnesia may be ordered to help eliminate the barium.
3. Repeat test is ordered if visualization was hindered by barium or stool.
4. Test is interpreted by radiologist.

DOUBLE AIR CONTRAST OF COLON (DOUBLE CONTRAST BARIUM ENEMA)

Description: A more accurate barium enema examination in which air is pumped into the rectum to more clearly delineate the walls of the colon.

Preparation: Refer to barium examination.

Patient teaching:
1. Patient's lower bowel is filled by enema with barium and air pumped from a bulb.
2. Abdominal cramps or discomfort may be experienced along with a strong urge to defecate.

3. Enema should not be expelled until films are completed.
4. Patient will experience more tipping and turning on table than with the barium enema.
5. Examination takes one to two hours.

Implementation: Refer to barium enema examination.

Evaluation: Refer to barium enema examination.

COLONOSCOPY

Description: An endoscopic examination in which the anal insertion of a fiberoptic colonoscope is used to demonstrate abnormalities of the colon and ileocecal valve, such as bleeding sites, ulceration, or polyps. This direct visualization allows photographs, biopsies, excisions, and fulguration.

Preparation:
1. Patient's signed permission is necessary.
2. Diet change prior to test is ordered by physician.
3. Specific directions for cleansing the colon are given by the physician.
4. Premedication is ordered by physician.
5. Physician should be consulted concerning diet and insulin for diabetic patients.
6. Can be done before or three days after barium studies.

Patient teaching:
1. Patient lies on left side with knees drawn up to the abdomen.
2. Flexible tube is lubricated and inserted into the rectum and advanced so that the physician can examine the colon and take tissue specimens for biopsy.
3. Physician asks patient to take deep breaths or change position as the colonoscope is advanced.
4. Discomfort and possible cramping may be experienced during this test.
5. Examination takes one to two hours.

Implementation: Patient is transported by wheelchair, if
                       ambulatory; otherwise, send by cart.

Evaluation: The findings are evaluated by the
                       gastroenterologist.

LARYNGIOGRAM

Description: A laryngoscope and the oral administration of
                      radiopaque, iodine-containing material are used
                      to demonstrate abnormalities, such as lesions,
                      tumors, or dysfunctions of the vocal cords,
                      epiglottis, base of the tongue, and uvula.

Preparation: 1. Iodine allergies (seafood) or allergic reaction
                         to previous iodine tests should be reported
                         to physician and radiology department.
                      2. Preparation is not required.

Patient teaching: 1. Local anesthetic spray is administered.
                      2. Laryngoscope is passed into the larynx, and
                         dye is instilled.
                      3. Patient is asked to phonate or say, "Three,
                         three, three."
                      4. Patient experiences fullness in the throat,
                         but there is little discomfort.
                      5. Examination takes about 15 minutes.

Implementation: Patient is sent to radiology via wheelchair if
                      ambulatory; otherwise, send by cart.

Evaluation: 1. Allergic reaction is possible if the patient is
                         allergic to iodine-containing materials. It's
                         rarely severe, but should be considered.
                      2. Patient may not take food or fluids until the
                         swallow reflex returns, usually a very brief
                         time; otherwise, no special care is required.
                      3. Test is interpreted by radiologist.

PULMONARY FUNCTION TESTS (PFT)

Description:	A respiratory examination in which a series of breathing tests demonstrate abnormalities of the lungs, such as obstructive or restrictive lung disease, and provide evaluation of pulmonary status preoperatively. 1. Complete scan consists of: • FVC—functional vital capacity, • MVC—maximum vital capacity, • DL Co—single-breath diffusion carbon monoxide, and • TLC—Total lung capacity. 2. Pre-op scan consists of FVC and MVC.
Preparation:	1. Loose clothing should be worn during testing. Belts and other constrictive clothing are removed. 2. Measures aimed at removing secretions, such as suctioning or chest physical therapy, should be performed prior to the test. 3. Interfering condition is a thoracostomy.
Patient teaching:	1. Patient is seated in a chair next to computerized spirometer. 2. Nose clip is placed on the patient's nose and a rubber mouthpiece is placed in the mouth. 3. Patient is asked to breathe normally, then to inhale and exhale deeply, and finally to breathe as rapidly as possible. 4. Bronchodilators may be used to compare pulmonary measurements if patient's written permission has been given. 5. Blood gases may also be drawn at this time. 6. Fatigue or shortness of breath may be experienced, depending on the patient's physical condition. 7. Examination takes 15 minutes to one hour.
Implementation:	Patient is transported *via wheelchair only.* Accurate results cannot be obtained with the patient on a cart.
Evaluation:	Test is interpreted by a chest physiologist.

PNEUMOENCEPHALOGRAM

Description: An X-ray examination in which the injection of air or gas into the spinal column is used to demonstrate abnormalities, such as displacement by tumor or abscess or enlargement with hydrocephalus, of the ventricles and subarachnoid space. Rarely used as there are safer tests with fewer side effects that provide essentially the same information, such as computerized tomography.

Preparation:
1. Preparation other than the following is specifically ordered.
2. Patient's signed permission must be obtained.
3. Premedication is usually ordered by physician.
4. Meal prior to test is omitted.
5. Physician should be consulted regarding diet and insulin for diabetic patients.
6. Increased spinal fluid pressure can be an interfering condition.

Patient teaching:
1. Lumbar spine area is cleansed and a local anesthetic is administered.
2. Patient assumes a knee-chest position.
3. Radiologist inserts a needle between two vertebrae in the lumbar region of the patient's spine.
4. Spinal fluid is removed and air is injected to fill the ventricles and subarachnoid space.
5. Films are taken in several series with the patient in various positions on the table.
6. Injected air in the ventricles will be absorbed and replaced by spinal fluid after a day or two.
7. Examination takes two to four hours.

Implementation:
1. Premedicate as ordered "on call."
2. Patient is sent to radiology *per cart only* with his chart and signed permission.

Evaluation:
1. Test is canceled if increased spinal fluid pressure is present.

2. Puncture site is inspected for leakage of cerebrospinal fluid or edema, which, if found, are reported to the physician.
3. Vital signs and neurological status are monitored according to this schedule:
   - q15min for one hour,
   - q30min for next two hours,
   - qh for next four hours, then
   - q4h if stable.
4. Patient lies prone six to eight hours after the test and is logrolled side, back, side q 2 hours to hasten absorption of the air. Bedrest is maintained until the following day, and activity is then resumed gradually.
5. Normal diet is resumed unless otherwise ordered.
6. Fluids are encouraged unless contraindicated.
7. Side effects include headaches, nausea, vomiting, and tinnitus.
8. Test is interpreted by radiologist.

MYELOGRAM

Description: An X-ray examination in which injection into the subarachnoid space is used to demonstrate abnormalities of the spinal column, such as tumors, vertebral fractures, disc ruptures, or meningeal inflammation.

Preparation:
1. Iodine allergies (seafood) or allergic reactions to previous iodine tests should be reported to the physician and radiology department.
2. Patient's signed permission is necessary.
3. Preparation is specifically ordered by physician.
4. Does *not* have to be NPO from midnight.
5. Premedication is usually ordered by the physician.
6. Physician should be consulted concerning diet and insulin for diabetic patients.
7. Spinal tray is needed for this procedure.
8. Increased spinal fluid pressure is an interfering condition.

Patient teaching: 1. Lumbar spine area is cleansed and a local anesthetic administered.
2. Patient assumes a knee-chest position or lies prone with a pillow under the pelvic region.
3. Radiologist inserts a needle between two vertebrae in the lumbar region of the spine.
4. Spinal fluid is removed and contrast dye injected.
5. Examination takes one to two hours.
6. Films are taken at intervals with the patient in prone position on a tilt table which is maneuvered into various positions. Patient is held securely by foot and shoulder supports.
7. Examination takes one to two hours.

Implementation: 1. Premedicate as ordered "on call."
2. Patient is sent to radiology *per cart* only with his chart, permission, and spinal tray.
3. A nurse or physician should accompany unstable or emergency patients.

Evaluation: 1. Test is canceled if increased spinal fluid pressure is present.
2. Allergic reactions should be considered if the patient is allergic to iodine-containing materials. Report to the physician nausea, vomiting, respiratory distress, flushing, or urticaria.
3. Puncture site is inspected for edema or leakage of cerebrospinal fluid. Report any to the physician.
4. Vital signs and neurological status are monitored according to this schedule:
   - q15min for one hour,
   - q30min for next two hours,
   - qh for next four hours, then
   - q4h if stable.
5. Patient lies prone six to eight hours after the test and is logrolled side, back, side q2h to hasten absorption of the dye. Bedrest is maintained until the following day, and activity is then resumed gradually.

6. Urine specific gravity should be taken after each voiding until it returns to pretest level to ascertain that the dye is being eliminated.
7. Current diet is resumed unless otherwise ordered.
8. Fluids are encouraged unless contraindicated.
9. Most common side effects are headaches or neck stiffness, which may last a few hours or days.
10. Test is interpreted by the radiologist.

ELECTROENCEPHALOGRAM (EEG)

Description: Electric impulses are recorded on paper by a machine called an electroenccphalogram. Electrodes are attached to the scalp with colloiden. The test can localize surface brain lesions, such as scars, tumors, blood clots, and abscesses, and also determinc the presence of epilepsy.

Preparation:
1. Sedatives are generally withheld up to the night before.
2. Anticonvulsant medication may be withheld by physician order.
3. On the day of the test, patient should take no stimulants or depressants, such as coffee, tea, cola, or alcoholic beverages.
4. Patient should not fast prior to the test.
5. Hair should be washed and free of oil or dirt that may interfere with the electrode contact.

Patient teaching:
1. Patient lies on a table in a darkened room and is asked to close his eyes and rest.
2. Electrodes are placed on the scalp.
3. Patient should be instructed that an EEG picks up impulses from the brain. It does *not* send electricity to the brain. There is no danger of electric shock.
4. During the tests, the patient may be asked to hyperventilate or perform simple mental activity.

Implementation: Patient is sent for EEG via wheelchair if ambulatory; otherwise, send by cart with chart.

Evaluation:
1. Patient may resume pre-examination activities.
2. Results interpreted by neurologist.

BONE MARROW BIOPSY

Description: A sternal needle is inserted through the bone cortex into the marrow space to withdraw 1-2 ml of marrow. This test is used to diagnose most blood dyscrasias, including aplastic anemia, leukemia, pernicious anemia, and thrombocytopenia. Examination of the bone marrow reveals the number, size, and shape of red cells, white cells, and platelets in their various developmental stages.

Preparation:
1. Signed patient permission must be obtained.
2. An order for sedation or analgesic may be ordered by physician.

Patient teaching:
1. Since the iliac crest is the site, patient will lie on his side with knees drawn up to abdomen.
2. Area for insertion is cleansed, and local anesthetic administered.
3. Needle is inserted into bone area, and bone biopsy is obtained.
4. Some pressure or slight pain may be experienced.
5. Sterile dressing is applied to insertion site and remains on for 24 hours.
6. Patient may shower after 24 hours.
7. Slight soreness of lower back may be experienced up to three to four days following procedure.
8. Examination will take 15 to 30 minutes.

Implementation:
1. Premedication given as ordered "on call."
2. Biopsy is done in room, and patient should be positioned on side.

3. Biopsy tray in room in advance of test.
4. Specimen is sent to laboratory in a jar containing preservative.

Evaluation:

1. Area is checked q4h for 24 hours for bleeding and infection.
2. Patient may resume diet and activity after test.
3. Dressing may be removed after 24 hours if no complications.
4. Test interpreted by physician.

RADIOISOTOPE "SCANS"

Description: Diagnostically, radioisotopes can be used as tracers. A scanner measures the uptake of the radioisotope. Radioisotopes are used to locate tumors and lesions of the brain, kidneys, liver, lungs, periosteum, and bones.

Preparation: No specific preparation is required.

Patient teaching:

1. Patient is given a tracer dose of appropriate radioisotope either orally or by injection.
2. Radioisotopes are given in extremely small doses; therefore, the body absorbs a minimal amount of radiation.
3. Depending on the organ being scanned, the isotope may be given one to two hours before scanning so the isotope will be absorbed.
4. The patient lies on a table under a scanner.
5. Patient will be asked to lie still. The scanner moves over the area to be studied.

Implementation: Patient is sent to nuclear medicine via wheelchair if ambulatory; otherwise, send by cart.

Evaluation:

1. Patient may resume pretest orders.
2. Fluids are encouraged unless contraindicated.
3. Results are interpreted by radiologist.

ULTRASOUND

Description:	A noninvasive examination in which high-frequency sound waves are used to demonstrate abnormalities, such as cysts, tumors, and abscesses of organs or tissues with various densities.

Preparation:
1. Preparation depends on the organ to be studied and should be ordered by physician.
2. Physician should be consulted concerning diet and insulin for diabetic patients. These patients should be scheduled first.
3. Obesity and barium studies within three days can interfere with ultrasound.
4. Patient should empty bladder prior to test.

Patient teaching:
1. Patient lies on the examination table. The technician puts mineral oil on the abdomen to promote good skin contact. As a probe is moved across the skin, an image of the internal organ is then visualized and photographed.
2. Test causes no discomfort, except in the case of a full bladder during pelvic ultrasound.
3. Examination takes up to one hour.

Implementation: Patient is sent to ultrasound via wheelchair if ambulatory; otherwise, send by cart.

Evaluation:
1. Special care after test is not required.
2. Repeat test is ordered if visualization was hindered by previous barium studies.
3. Test is interpreted by the radiologist.

COMPUTERIZED TOMOGRAPHY

Description:	An X-ray examination in which radiologic films and a computer are used to demonstrate abnormalities of the head or body. Less risky than invasive procedures such as pneumoencephalography or angiography.

Preparation: 1. Iodine allergies (seafood) or allergic reactions
to previous iodine tests should be reported
to the physician and radiology department if
the test is ordered with IV contrast
materials.
2. Restless patients may require sedation as
ordered by the physician.
3. Barium from previous tests must be
removed prior to a body scan.
4. Barium studies done within three days prior
to or scheduled for within three days after
scan may interfere with test.
5. Body scan may require use of oral or IV
administration of iodine-containing material.
If IV contrast dye is used, it is administered
slowly. The body part to be examined is
centered within the tunnel. Some body
examinations require a delay between the
administration of the oral contrast medium
and the initiation of the test.

Patient teaching: 1. The examination room contains a large, box-
like structure enclosing the X-ray tube and
scanning equipment. The X-ray tube moves
in a circular fashion, sending radiation
through the head or body. This radiation is
measured on the other side by receptors, fed
into a computer, and visualized on a screen.
2. Discomfort results only from being required
to lie still for an extended period.
3. Examination takes 45 minutes to one hour.

Implementation: 1. Patient is sent to radiology with the patient
chart via wheelchair if ambulatory;
otherwise, send by cart.
2. Professional staff should accompany
unstable or emergency patients.

Evaluation: 1. Allergic reaction should be considered if the
patient is allergic to iodine-containing
materials. Report to the physician nausea,
vomiting, respiratory distress, flushing, or
urticaria.
2. IV injection site is inspected for signs of
infiltration, such as redness, swelling, pain,

or a burning sensation. Apply ice to the infiltrated site and notify physician.

3. Hypotension may occur in some patients if IV contrast dye is used.
4. Urine specific gravity should be taken after each voiding until it returns to pretest level, to assure that the dye is being eliminated.
5. Oral contrast dye may cause diarrhea.
6. Fluids are encouraged unless contraindicated.
7. Repeat body scan is necessary if visualization was hindered by previous barium studies.
8. Test is interpreted by the radiologist.

Surgical diagnosis

Surgical intervention may be required to detect cancer, to confirm diagnosis, or to determine the extent of the cancer. During this time of diagnosis, the patient and family are usually anxious or apprehensive. Nursing care in this phase emphasizes appropriate patient education, comfort, precise preparation for the selected surgical procedure, and emotional support of the patient, family, and friends.

A wide variety of procedures can be used in surgical intervention to confirm the presence of cancer or to aid in making a positive diagnosis. Surgery is an invasive technique that requires adequate patient preparation, careful attention to details of care before, during, and following surgery, and assessment to detect complications and the patient's physical and psychological response to the procedure. Specific care measures are predicated on the type of surgery, the type of anesthesia used, the patient's pre-existing condition, and response to the procedure. The patient may undergo one or a combination of several surgical diagnostic procedures.

TYPES OF SURGICAL PROCEDURES

Biopsy: Three types of biopsies are needle, excisional, and incisional. Each type is performed to obtain a tissue sample for laboratory analysis. A sample of a suspicious area, node, or tumor is sent to the laboratory and examined microscopically to determine the presence of benign or malignant cells.

Scope: Mediastinoscopy and bronchoscopy are two of the many procedures that allow direct visualization of a specific body area. Bronchoscopy allows the physician to visualize the tracheobronchial tree. Mediastinoscopy allows visualization of the paratracheal and tracheobronchial areas and lymph nodes in the region. Performed with either local or general anesthesia, depending on physician preference and evaluation of the patient, these procedures also are used to obtain specimens for laboratory analysis, for pathologic evaluation, and to determine the extent of spread in the body region.

Exploratory laparotomy: Surgery is performed to aid in confirmation of diagnosis. The surgeon defines and isolates suspected abnormal cell growth and determines whether a tumor mass is present, its size, and also obtains a specimen for analysis.

Staging laparotomy: Surgery is performed to locate the primary tumor and the extent of its involvement, including lymph node involvement, and findings are used by the physician to determine the appropriate treatment plan.

Progression of cancer

Cancer invades the body in different patterns of spread that can now be projected on the basis of scientific observation of the course cancer has taken in people who have previously been treated. When cancer is diagnosed, it is necessary to determine the type of cancer and its grade through microscopic analysis, the primary site of the cancer, and the extent of invasion. Exploratory surgery for staging and grading of cancers thus provides information needed to initiate a medical plan of treatment specific to the individual patient's cancer.

CLASSIFICATION OF TUMORS

In addition to histologic determination of the type of cancer cell, tumors are staged and graded. The mechanisms of spread to other body parts, such as through regional lymph nodes, and the propensity of certain types of tumors to extend and invade other body tissues are known through observations of many patients over time. Current methods of clinical staging and grading are based on findings from the total diagnostic workup. Appropriate therapy is then determined by the classification of a particular type of cancer, which indicates the type of tumor, the extent of spread, and thus the patient's prognosis.

The *stage* of tumor growth refers to the maturity of the cancer cell and its differentiation. The International Classification System for Staging is as follows:

   0. carcinoma in situ
   I. limited to tumor,
   II. tumor with local lymph node extension,
   III. tumor with extension beyond primary site or organ, and
   IV. extension to distant body regions.

The TNM classification was developed by the American Joint Committee for Cancer Staging and End Results Reporting. In this system, T refers to the primary tumor, and T_1, T_2, T_3, and T_4 refer to progressive increases in tumor size and involvement. N refers to regional lymph node involvement, N_0 no lymph nodes involved, N_1 one lymph node

TABLE 3-1 GENERAL GUIDELINES FOR STAGING
AND GRADING OF CANCER*

Stage	T = primary tumor	N = regional lymph node involvement	M = distant metastases
I	T_1	N_0	M_0
	Mass is limited to origin; lesion is operable and resectable with only local involvement; no nodal and vascular spread. Chance of survival: 70–90%		
II	T_2	N_1	M_0
	Clinical evidence shows local spread to surrounding tissue and first station lymph nodes; lesion is operable and resectable, but there would be uncertainty as to completeness of removal; there may be evidence of microinvasion into capsule and lymphatics. Chance of survival: 5–50%		
III	T_3	N_2	M_0
	There is extensive primary disease with fixation to deeper structure and invasion into bone and lymph nodes; lesion is operable but not resectable, and gross disease is left behind. Chance of survival: 5–20%		
IV	T_4	N_3	M_+
	There is evidence of distance metastases beyond local site of organ; the lesion is inoperable. Chance of survival: <5%		

*From *Clinical Oncology for Medical Students and Physicians: A Multidisciplinary Approach.* 5th ed. Rochester, NY: University of Rochester School of Medicine/Dentisty, 1978.

involved, N_2 more than one lymph node involved, and N_3 and N_4 refer to degrees of regional lymph node involvement. M refers to metastases; M_0 means no metastases, and M_+ means distant metastases.

Table 3-1 provides information about general guidelines for staging and grading of cancers. It should be emphasized that various specialty medical groups have different classification systems and each system pertains to characteristics of different tumor types and different patterns of metastases. Efforts are under way to develop classification systems that could be used for staging and grading each type of cancer according to its location in the body and usual pattern of extension.

Planning nursing care

There are eight major areas the nurse incorporates into the plan of care:

1. The intended surgery and purpose of the planned procedure.

2. The nurse must ensure that all preoperative bloodwork, urinalysis, X-rays, electrocardiogram, and sputum specimens have been completed, with the results noted on the patient's chart, and abnormal results appropriately reported to the physician.

3. The patient is required to sign a consent form. The physician who will perform the surgery is responsible for obtaining the patient's informed written consent. The nurse must make sure that the signed consent is in order and on the patient's chart prior to administering any preoperative medications.

The patient's written consent must be an informed consent, which means that the patient or legally responsible adult has been told of and is able to comprehend the intended surgical procedure, possible risks, and complications.

4. Often a preoperative visit by the anesthesiologist is scheduled so that the patient can discuss the type of anesthesia and ask questions. It is important that the nurse know the intended plan and appropriately reinforce the information that the anesthesiologist gives the patient. The nurse must know the effects of general anesthesia and be prepared to answer any additional questions from the patient.

5. The patient will usually be NPO after midnight. In some cases, the patient may be allowed a clear liquid breakfast and then be NPO.

6. The nurse should know about any *pre-existing conditions the patient has, such as diabetes, previous cardiac condition, and medications taken previously and currently.*

7. The nurse should know of any previous medication allergies. In obtaining the nursing history, previous reactions to a specific drug, specific information about the type of reactions, such as rash, nausea, vomiting, rhinitis, or congestion, are ascertained. Once a patient's immune system has been sensitized to an antigen from a certain drug, the next time he or she receives that particular drug, it could produce an anaphylactic reaction, which is a life-threatening situation.

8. The nurse must know the purpose, potential drug interactions, and side effects of each preoperative medication, such as meperidine (Demerol), morphine sulphate, atropine, or diazepam (Valium). The nurse administers the medication correctly to ensure the desired sedative effects, maintain patient safety, and observe any undesirable reactions before the patient leaves for the operating room.

PREOPERATIVE TEACHING

The nurse provides emotional support and preoperative teaching for patients and families during preoperative care. In many hospitals, the physician, the anesthesiologist, and the nurse form a team to inform and teach the patient and family about the anticipated surgery. Many patient-education tools are available. Booklets can be used and in many hospitals closed-circuit television is used for patient education programs. Preoperative group teaching sessions with slides, movies, and general discussion are also effective. The nurse should be up-to-date with regard to what resources are available for preoperative teaching and should use them to supplement and expand individualized patient education.

TEACHING PLAN

The nurse must first assess the patient's previous knowledge about the procedure. Then, in discussion with the patient, determine his or her perception of local or general anesthesia and of the intended surgical procedure. Instruct the patient as appears necessary from your discussion and answer his questions. Show the patient techniques of an effective cough, deep breathing, and special breathing exercises and have the patient demonstrate these exercises.

The following is a guide to important areas of patient instruction. Instructions such as these should be used both in conference with the patient and family to review or recall the scheduled events and to reduce their fear of the unknown.

Patient Instructions: Operative Care

PREOPERATIVE

1. Following surgery, correct coughing to remove secretions and deep breathing to expand the lungs are essential, since you have had anesthesia and also are not exercising as you would normally.
   - *Coughing:* To cough correctly, take a deep breath and cough, using your abdominal muscles.
   - *Diaphragmatic breathing:* Place your hand on your stomach and exhale through your mouth. Feel your stomach tighten and sink. Inhale, then relax stomach and allow stomach and hand to rise. Keep upper chest still, then exhale.
   - *Lateral costal breathing:* First position yourself, either sitting or lying, and place hands on ribs. Exhale and press on ribs at the same time. Inhale and release pressure on ribs.
2. You may be given a sedative (sleeping pill) to help you sleep well. Because the sedative may make you feel groggy, the side rails on your bed will be raised, and you should call your nurse if you need to get up during the night.
3. You may not eat any foods or drink any fluids, including water, after midnight.
4. Because you will not eat or drink, a special tube may be inserted into a vein for intravenous infusion (IV), either in your room the night before surgery or in the operating room in the morning.
5. As a precaution to prevent infection, the area of your body where the surgical incision will be made may be shaved and you may be asked to take a shower, using a special soap, before surgery.

MORNING OF SURGERY

6. The nurse will try to awaken you early to allow you time to shower (and shave) and get prepared before surgery.
7. The nurse will take your temperature, blood pressure, and check your heart rate and respirations.
8. You will be asked to remove dentures, contact lenses, or any other artificial devices.
9. Your wedding ring will be taped to your finger, but all other jewelry, money, credit cards, or valuables should be given to a family member or to the nurse to be locked up for safekeeping while you are out of your room.
10. You will be asked to put on a hospital gown.
11. Just before leaving for the operating room, you will be asked to urinate (empty your bladder).

12. Then the nurse will give you your preoperative medication, either an injection or a pill. You will be asked to remain in bed, and the side rails will be raised. You may begin to feel drowsy. As your body relaxes, you may experience a dryness in your mouth.
13. An operating room orderly will arrive in your room with a cart to take you to the operating room.
14. While you are having your surgery, your family and friends may wait in the surgical waiting lounge.
15. After your surgery is completed, you will be taken to the recovery room until you are fully awake and ready to return to your hospital room or to the intensive care unit.
16. Once you return to your hospital bed, the nurse will frequently check your blood pressure, heart rate, and respiration.
17. The nurse will assist you in turning from side to side, coughing, and deep breathing.
18. Initially you will not be allowed to get out of bed, except when assisted by your nurse.
19. If you are uncomfortable, the nurse will give you a pain medication ordered by your physician to keep you comfortable.

SUMMARY

Once a firm diagnosis is made, the nursing plan of care must incorporate aspects of assisting the patient to cope with family responses, financial considerations, absence from work, and possible future change in body image and sometimes in life goals. At this time, the patient is simultaneously confronted with a threatened future, with possible change in life-style, and with choices for future treatment.

BIBLIOGRAPHY

American Joint Committee for Cancer Staging and End Results Reporting. MANUAL FOR STAGING OF CANCER. New York: American Cancer Society, 1978.

Bearhs OH and Myers MH, eds. MANUAL FOR STAGING OF CANCER. Philadelphia: Lippincott, 1983.

Bogolin L and Harris JE, eds. Meeting the immunological challenge—Rush Presbyterian-St. Luke's Medical Center symposium. HEART LUNG 9:643, 1980.

Cazalas MW. NURSING AND THE LAW. Rockville, Md: Aspen, 1979.

DIAGNOSTIC AND PROCEDURE PAMPHLET. Evanston, Ill: Evanston Hospital Corporation.

DIAGNOSTICS. Springhouse, Pa: Intermed, 1981.

THE EVANSTON HOSPITAL PRE-OPERATIVE TEACHING BOOKLET. Evanston, Ill: Evanston Hospital Corporation.

Fruth R. Anaphylaxis and drug reactions: Guidelines for detection and care. HEART LUNG 9:662, 1980.

Hemelt MD and Mackert ME. DYNAMICS OF LAW IN NURSING AND HEALTH CARE. Reston, Va: Reston, 1978.

PROGRAM GUIDE, PATIENT EDUCATION TELEVISION. Evanston, Ill: Evanston Hospital Corporation.

Rosai J and Ackerman LV. THE PATHOLOGY OF TUMORS. New York: American Cancer Society, 1978.

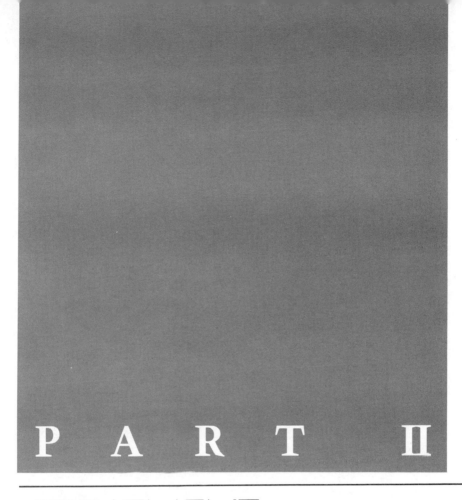

PART II

TREATMENT

4
SURGERY

MICHELLE A. McCLANAHAN, RN, BS

The plan of treatment of the cancer patient may involve several oncology specialists from various health-care disciplines. Among the physicians who may care for the patient, either in direct care or consultation, are the patient's personal physician, a surgeon, radiation oncologist, and medical oncologist, depending on the type of treatment selected.

The patient may also be cared for by a number of nurses in different specialty areas in sequence or concurrently. Care may necessitate being transferred from one patient care unit to another. Thus the care givers must plan for effective communication that promotes continuity in the patient's care. Continuity is necessary to prevent further disruption in the patient's changing status.

Oncology patients may experience many physical and psychological changes during treatment of their illness. They may undergo either one form or a combination of treatment approaches within a short time. Many cancer patients feel anger and guilt secondary to delay in seeking medical attention for their symptoms. Many face an uncertain future under the threat of death. In some institutions, a clinical nurse psychiatric specialist may assist the patient and nurses to effectively work through these physical and psychological changes.

Physical changes the patient experiences may result from the effects of cancer on the body and from the various treatment modalities. A patient may have surgery with consequent body disfigurement or altered perceptions of sexuality. Chemotherapy may cause severe nausea, vomiting, loss of hair, fatigue, or other symptoms. The patient may experience frustration because of the disruption in his or her life-style, interruption of work or leisure, and in relationships. Physical changes thus are entwined with psychological changes that must be considered in your comprehensive plan for the patient's care.

A major nursing role is to ease the patient's adjustment to treatment-induced illness, body changes, and emotional concerns about the diagnosis, prognosis, and options for the future. In this process of adjustment, the patient's coping mechanisms are a key element. Recognizing that the patients' participation in planning and implementing their care will influence their ability to cope with cancer and its implications, encourages patients to take an active role. Other health professionals can also help the patients adjust.

In many settings, personnel who care for cancer patients are organized in a multidisciplinary health-care team. The team includes surgeons, radiation and medical oncologists, oncology nurses, nutritionists, and social workers. All these caregivers participate in regular review and update of the patient's progress. Even though patients may be transferred back and forth from inpatient to outpatient status, if they are in the care of a health-care team, they have the benefit of continuity in their care by a team with whom they are acquainted.

Patients may also benefit from several other programs that are usually part of an organized cancer-care-center approach. Pain management programs assist patients in pain therapy. Self-help support groups have been established for patients and families to meet on a regular basis. Formal education programs are often an integral part of community efforts to help patients and their families in coping with the diagnosis of cancer and its implications.

Care of the oncology patient goes beyond the traditional definition of treatment and includes meeting the challenge that results from the course of treatment, and the patient's prognosis and response to the physical and psychological changes resulting from the diagnosis of cancer. In every instance, the positive aspects of cure and care are emphasized, and the patient is given the maximum opportunity to be part of the treatment team that plans and implements care.

Below and in the following chapters, specific forms of treatment are outlined. Though each is presented separately, in practice, patients may receive combinations of treatment forms, depending on their status.

A majority of cancer patients are treated by surgical resection. Of the 55 percent of patients treated by surgery, 40 percent have surgery as the sole treatment modality. Frequently, the nurse who cares for the patient at the time of initial diagnosis of cancer continues with the patient through surgery. Patients may return to surgery if it becomes necessary to control the disease, for reconstruction, to relieve complications, or as a palliative measure. For these patients, the patient-nurse bond that forms is vital to quality care as the patient goes through emotional and physical insult.

When you function as a primary nurse for the surgical oncology patient, you acquire valuable knowledge of the patient that enables realistic, successful implementation of the nursing process. You can follow the patient during outpatient care and through future hospitalizations for further treatments. During this often confusing time period for the patient, you can provide a valuable stable link to the total care process.

This consistency in care by a designated primary nurse allows the patient to form a relationship with the nurse based on trust and familiarity that can greatly influence hospitalization and outcomes of treatment. Through the phases of surgery, you prepare patients for each successive event and help them learn self-care. Teaching the patient how to care for a colostomy and helping a patient who has had a mastectomy regain arm movement by exercising are nursing functions that culminate in the patient's independence in self-care.

Preoperative Nursing Care

The purpose of surgery for the oncology patient is cure or control of cancer. As a result of surgical intervention, the patient may experience body disfigurement or functional loss of an organ or body system. Preoperative nursing thus deals with the patient's responses to diagnosis and the treatment interventions. In this part of the nursing process, assessment of the patient's physical and emotional status provides essential data for planning the immediate and longer-range nursing measures. How the patient deals with the preoperative situation aids in planning for later phases of care. The patient is informed prior to surgery of possible disfigurement or loss of some body function. So, in addition to preoperative anxiety about the surgery and the potential prognosis, the patient may have to face a change in body image. It is important for you to accurately assess the patient's level of anxiety in preoperative teaching. Some patients may be able to understand the implications of surgery and want information about their postoperative rehabilitation, and other patients may not be able to focus beyond the immediate moment.

Patients' ability to comprehend information about surgery and its potential outcomes is influenced by their physical status. Pre-existing conditions, such as respiratory or cardiac disease, may reduce the patients' energy level and decrease their reserves to cope with the stress of the current diagnosis and treatment. Patients with complicated surgery, such as thoracotomy, or multisystem illnesses may require more intense and complex care before and after surgery. These patients may go to an intensive care unit postoperatively. The nurse needs to explain well beforehand how an intensive care unit differs from the regular room and why there is need for close surveillance of them. The patient who has not had previous experience with an ICU, either personally or through a family member's hospitalization, will need particularly sensitive teaching. A tour of the unit may be arranged to assist in the preparation. At the time of transfer from ICU, every attempt should be made to return the patient to the previous unit and the primary nurse in order to maximize the benefits of consistency in nursing care. It is also important in a multidisciplinary approach that all care givers unite and share information concerning findings and the operative plan so that they all have accurate information.

NURSING MEASURES

1. Assess the patient's situation including the status of diagnosis, the purposes of surgery, and the uncertainties he or she will face.
2. Determine the effects the particular type of surgery to be performed may have on the patient's body image and functional body processes.
3. Assess the potential complications and special care measures the patient's pre-existing physical status requires, including illnesses resolved and those under current therapy.
4. Assess the patient's level of anxiety about the diagnosis, surgery, and the outcomes of surgery and the family responses to the patient's illness.
5. Determine the patient's level of understanding about the surgery and the procedures and environment to be experienced in perioperative and immediate postoperative care.
6. Assess the patient's ability to deal with information.
7. Provide the patient with information according to assessment of the capability to comprehend and deal with knowledge of treatment. Plan treatment to accommodate the patient's ability to focus on present and future events.

8. Ensure that the patient and family understand the events of the surgical procedure and possible outcomes.
9. Ensure that the nursing care plan appropriately coordinates care provided by other caregivers and that the plan is commonly understood and supported.

PERIOPERATIVE CARE

The surgeon determines an operative plan after reviewing the patient's history, findings of the physical examination, and diagnostic tests. As a member of the patient's team of caregivers, the primary nurse is informed of the operative plan and follows through with nursing care as indicated by the surgeon's plan and nursing assessment findings. Good communication among members of the patient-care team is a key element in the effectiveness of the total management of the surgical oncology patient.

Advances in surgical technique have been made possible with increased knowledge of tumor cell physiology. Approximately two-thirds of a tumor's growth cycle (cell divisions) occurs before it is clinically detectable.

In the excision of a tumor mass, it's necessary to remove a portion of the surrounding normal tissue, to eliminate the possibility of residual tumor cells at the excision site. The greater the infiltration of tumor cells to tissue outside of the mass, the wider the excision or the more radical the procedure becomes. During excision, extreme care is taken to work from the periphery toward the tumor and to remove the mass gingerly, with its surrounding tumor bed intact. It's often necessary also to remove regional lymph nodes, because tumor cells disseminate via the lymphatic system.

REPEAT SURGERY

Positive metastasis to another area may necessitate repeat surgery. This is done either to control metastases, as in the patient with a mastectomy who undergoes a thoracotomy, or to control symptoms resulting from extension of the cancer. In these cases, the surgeon ascertains if the spread is confined or widely spread to more than one area before the patient is on the operating room table.

RECONSTRUCTIVE SURGERY

Cancer patients may return to the hospital for reconstructive surgery. The procedures may be for either cosmetic or functional repair. For example, the mastectomy patient may desire a breast implant or augmentation, procedures that can be done at the time of the initial mastectomy or several months later. Some ostomy patients may have had a temporary colostomy and will return several weeks later for a "takedown" or closure of the colostomy. The patient's physical and psychological needs at the time of repeat surgery differ from what they were at the time of the initial surgical procedures. If reconstructive surgery is planned for cosmetic purposes, the patient may have high expectations, and you need to provide realistic information and emotional support.

Patients who come for another surgical procedure are usually familiar with the pre- and postoperative routines. They are subject, however, to increased risk from repeat general anesthesia, or they may be malnourished or anemic. It is best that such patients not undergo concomitant radiation or chemotherapy because these cause prolonged healing. Patients undergoing repeat surgery may have decreased reserves to handle stress. They may dread postoperative physical discomfort.

Postoperative Nursing Care

Postoperative needs of patients are influenced by the purpose of the surgery. If surgery is required to relieve symptoms such as an obstruction, to relieve pain, or to control bleeding, subsequent nursing care must be planned to meet the patient's special needs. Patients admitted for palliative procedures are usually in a debilitated physical condition as a result of the progress of the disease and previous treatment. Malnutrition may prolong the postoperative healing period. In some cases, there may be a delay in surgery until certain necessary corrective measures are taken—for example, blood transfusions in the patient who is seriously anemic.

POSTOPERATIVE NURSING CARE MEASURES
The following are the major components of nursing care of the postoperative patient.

1. *Pain control.* Initially, the patient will be NPO and require intramuscular injections with gradual change to oral pain medication. Adequate control of pain must be achieved for comfort and to allow for resumption of activity. Many cancer patients are afraid of becoming addicted to narcotics and the primary nurse needs to inform the patient that judicious use of pain control medication is helpful in recovery.

2. *Fluids and electrolyte balance.* The patient will have continuous intravenous therapy initially and then resume oral consumption. You must daily monitor electrolytes, intake and output, and weight.

3. *Estimated blood loss.* You should be aware of the patient's estimated blood loss (EBL) during the operation and monitor the hemoglobin and hematocrit as indications of actual blood loss.

4. *Nasogastric suction.* A majority of patients have a nasogastric tube in place, to be removed when bowel function returns.

5. *Nutritional support.* Gradual resumption of diet is started as active bowel sounds return. Depending on the patient's previous physical condition and type of surgery, hyperalimentation and/or tube feedings may be required.

6. *Activity.* The majority of patients are ambulated within a few hours after surgery. Exceptions are patients who have had a spinal anesthetic or were in a debilitated condition prior to surgery. Elderly patients require care in ambulation. Initially, ambulation may be complicated by tubes and IVs, often requiring two assisting persons.

7. *Respiratory care.* Most patients who have had a general anesthetic are given an incentive spirometer device to use on an hourly basis, 10 times per hour (Figure 4-1). If postoperative atelectasis develops, ultrasonic nebulizer treatments are initiated, and chest physical therapy may be added to the regimen. Some patients require high-humidity therapy in the initial few days to provide humidification of secretions and aid in mobilization of secretions.

8. *Wound care.* The treatment and type of wound care depends on the area involved and physician preference. You should check all dressings frequently and notify the doctor if significant drainage occurs, especially in the first few hours after the operation. Throughout the recovery period, continue to observe the suture line and note unusual swelling or redness and report purulent drainage.

    Following certain procedures, the wound may be left open for secondary closure. In these cases, the doctor usually orders some form of wound treatment, such as wet to dry dressing changes with Betadine or saline, wound irrigations, and packing to the area three to four times a day.

    If a wound infection develops, wound care is intensified. Cultures are obtained from the wound, and if the patient has an elevated temperature, blood and urine specimens are obtained for laboratory analysis. Information about the causative organism obtained from culture analysis is used to determine appropriate antibiotic therapy.

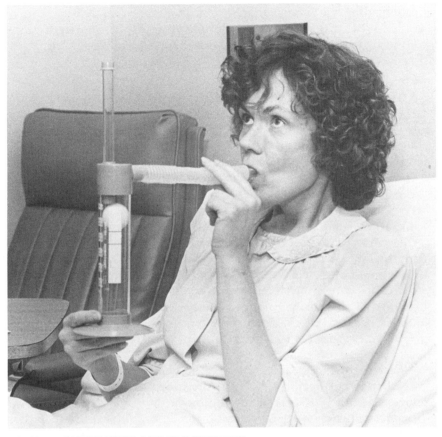

FIGURE 4 1. PATIENT USING INCENTIVE SPIROMETER.

POSTOPERATIVE COMPLICATIONS

The primary nurse must always be alert to the potential development of postoperative complications. Two major complications most frequently encountered are hemorrhage and wound infection.

Hemorrhage. The surgical dressing should be checked as soon as the patient returns to his or her room. The CBC is monitored because of possible internal bleeding along the suture line. Vital signs and urinary output are carefully monitored as they may indicate early hemorrhagic shock.

Wound infection. This complication develops several days after surgery. You can detect this complication by closely observing the suture line for increased redness, unusual swelling, or the presence of foul, purulent drainage accompanied by an increased temperature and increased WBC. Treatment may include systemic antibiotic therapy. Wound irrigation or frequent dressing changes may be needed.

CARE IN THE INTENSIVE CARE UNIT

After extensive surgery, the patient may be transferred to an intensive care unit for 24 to 48 hours. The type of surgical procedure, the patient's preoperative physical condition, or events that occur perioperatively determine the initial course of therapy.

Intensive care measures depend on the patient's postoperative status. Major body system functions are monitored, and adjunctive therapy may be required.

Cardiovascular and respiratory systems. The patient is placed on a cardiac monitor to observe the heart rhythm and to monitor potential arrhythmias. He or she may require mechanical ventilation and have an arterial line. If the patient has compromised cardiac status, a Swan-Ganz catheter is inserted before the operation.

Fluid and electrolyte balance. The patient may have several intravenous lines for fluid replacement and possible blood component therapy. A Foley catheter is inserted, usually in the operating room, to obtain accurate measurement of urinary output.

One or more surgical drains may be placed in the operative site. Immediately postoperatively, most drains are connected to a suction device. Both the character and amount of drainage are assessed, and the functioning of the drains is monitored according to their purpose and expected drainage.

NURSING CONSIDERATIONS

Being in intensive care and connected to tubes, wires, and machines can be frightening to the patient and family. Further, the ICU environment, with its 24-hour lights and noise, may not allow the patient adequate sleep. Although immediate family members are allowed to visit the patient for only brief intervals, in most hospitals a lounge for families and visitors is located near the unit. Before surgery, the patient and family should be informed of what to expect, and the family should be kept informed of the patient's status as care progresses. Family or friends may need advice or assistance during the patient's care, so you should maintain communication with them to assess their needs for information, expression of fear or worry, or assistance in planning how to accommodate their own and the patient's needs. Finally, both the patient and family should be prepared for the adjustment when the patient is transferred to another patient care area.

DISCHARGE PLANNING

Discharge planning begins on admission when the primary nurse determines the patient's support system outside of the hospital. The primary nurse and the physician need to work together with the patient to plan the time of discharge. Adequate time should be allowed for patient teaching of such matters as at-home colostomy care and tube feedings.

A multidisciplinary approach facilitates the patient's transition back to the home environment, particularly if the patient's care is complex. A social worker or a discharge planning coordinator are often part of the team. A discharge planning manual may be available as a reference and resource for you as you coordinate the patient's discharge.

Your first step in discharge planning is to assess the patient's care requirements. For example, a residual wound requires nursing assistance at home if a family member is unable or unwilling to assume responsibility for its care or if the patient lives alone. The following is a partial list of community services which illustrates the type of resources that may be used.

1. *Visiting Nurse Association (VNA).* This community service offers nursing care to assist the patient with further adjustment to an ostomy, continue with wound care or complicated dressing changes, or provide post-hospital assessment and follow-up. It is important to communicate care needs to the VNA nurse several days prior to the patient's discharge and to avoid untimely discharge on days the VNA service is not available. Continuity-of-care forms or discharge-planning forms provide a written report of the patient's status and care needs. Some VNAs have a post-hospitalization report that enables hospital nurses to follow the patient's progress after discharge.

2. *Meals on Wheels.* This community service delivers a hot meal once a day to patients who are unable to prepare their own food and live alone without family or friends' support. Frequently this service is arranged for elderly patients who need assistance. There is a small fee involved for the service, and arrangements need to be made prior to discharge, as there is usually a waiting list.

Several services are available through voluntary efforts:

3. *American Cancer Society.* The society may arrange for a hospital bed in the home for the terminal patient who desires to die at home, provide a variety of medical equipment and supplies, coordinate transportation for treatments or follow-up doctor's appointments, and provide information services, such as pamphlets, for use in patient teaching or supplemental information.

FIGURE 4-2 LARYNGECTOMY VOLUNTEER VISITING SERVICE

Patient's name _____ Date _____
Room no. _____ Home address _____
_____ City/Zip _____

Doctor:

Indicate below if you wish your patient to receive a pre- and/or postoperative visit from an American Cancer Society volunteer. The volunteer, also a laryngectomized person, may present the patient with a gift kit, including stoma bibs and literature encouraging the patient to learn esophageal speech.

Check as desired:

☐ Please arrange a preoperative visit.

☐ Please arrange a postoperative visit.

☐ Yes, present the kit when you visit _____ pre- _____ postoperatively.

☐ Omit literature.

_____
                                           Physician's signature/Date

Patient _____ referred to _____
                                           volunteer visitor

Hospital coordinator: When the physician completes this form, call a visitor assigned to your hospital, or the American Cancer Society office. Try to give the visitor as much advance notice as possible.

4. *Reach to Recovery.* This volunteer visiting service for mastectomy patients offers valuable assistance in selection of prosthesis, bras, and other measures. Volunteer visitors are women who have undergone a mastectomy, and efforts are made to match the volunteer with the patient according to age. Volunteers usually visit the patient in the hospital prior to discharge and again in the home environment. Arrangements with the service need to be made several days in advance.

5. *Lost Chord Club.* This is a voluntary organization composed of patients who have undergone a laryngectomy. Usually volunteers visit the patient before and after surgery, and there are regular group meetings that help in the adjustment process.

6. *Ostomy visitor.* Persons with an ostomy may volunteer their time to assist the new ostomy patient with support and practical advice.

A sample form for requesting volunteer laryngectomy service is shown in Figure 4-2.

SUMMARY

The primary nurse assesses the patient's discharge needs and resources available in the community and plans post-hospital care well in advance of discharge.

Health-care team members arrange for and assist the patient with plans for outpatient treatments and the further course of therapy.

The role of the primary nurse in the care of the surgical oncology patient requires competence in clinical skills, patience with teaching, and compassion. This care can be a satisfying and rewarding experience for the patient and the nurse. The bond that is formed between patient and nurse is long remembered. Unfortunately, many oncology patients return for further surgical intervention, and every effort should be made to reunite the patient with his nurse.

Selected Surgical Procedures

There are numerous procedures used in treatment for oncology patients—lymph node dissections and procedures for brain, bone, skin, or stomach cancer. Well-planned pre- and postoperative nursing care is required in all types of surgical intervention. Planning is more complex for patients who undergo extensive surgery that involves changing body image and learning to adapt to different ways of accommodating body functions. An example of such a patient is one who undergoes extensive surgery, such as removal of the uterus, bowel, and bladder with construction of a colostomy and possible urinary diversion (pelvic exenteration).

It is essential that you understand the planned surgical procedure and know your oncology patient's care requirements. Implications for nursing care differ for each surgical procedure. Some of the more frequently performed procedures are outlined in the following sections. These outlines, plus the sample nursing guidelines presented in the accompanying figures, provide a ready reference to key points to consider in nursing care.

BREAST (FIGURE 4-3—see page 80)

Procedures:
- *Radical mastectomy:* Includes removal of all breast tissue, axillary lymph nodes, and pectoral muscles.

Continued on page 84.

FIGURE 4-3 NURSING THE MASTECTOMY PATIENT

Potential problems	Nursing intervention or management	Outcome
• Shock secondary to: a. anesthesia b. blood loss	1. Check vital signs—BP, P, R (also skin color, temperature, LOC)—at least qh for four hours, then, if stable, q4h for one day, then qid for two days, then routine.	Documentation of VS, of initiated therapy for unstable patient.
	2. Include dressing check with VS, including posterior dressing because of gravity drainage.	Documentation of dressing changes.
	3. Assess drainage in Vacutainer. Evaluate amounts, depending on patient's general condition. If drainage > 100 cc/hr for two hours, notify surgeon.	Documentation of drainage, of initiated therapy if drainage > 100 cc.
	4. Maintain IV fluids (and blood if needed) until discontinued by physician pending CBC and tolerance of diet.	Maintenance of stable fluid and electrolytes.
• Pain due to surgery	1. Assess type and severity of pain, give medication when VS stable.	Patient able to complete exercises and ambulation with minimal discomfort.
	2. Instruct patient of availability and limits of pain medication.	
	3. Encourage medication at beginning of exercises.	
	4. Check functioning of drainage tubes; if nonfunctional, can cause increased pain.	
• Pneumonia secondary to: a. anesthesia b. hypoventilation c. immobility	1. Teach coughing and deep breathing and assess results q2h while awake, twice during night until A.M. of second POD.	Patient infection-free.
	2. Temperature q4h for one day, qid for two days (if elevated, q4h), then bid. Check qid for one day after drainage tubes are removed.	Documentation of elevated temperature, respiratory distress, that physician was notified.
	3. Activity a. Day of surgery—activity as ordered. b. First POD—up in chair & BRP qid. May ambulate as tolerated.	Patient freely ambulating, at least qid from second POD.

• Malfunction of drainage tubes	1. If Vacutainer used, check that tubes are collapsed when VS are taken.
	2. If uncollapsed:
	  a. Change bottle.
	  b. Milk tubing.
	  c. Check for air leaks (hissing).
	  d. Tape connections.
	  If above unsuccessful, notify physician.
	3. Change Vacutainer or Hemovac q shift and prn until tubes are removed. Chart output q shift. Keep bottle pinned to bed for safety.
	4. If tubes need to be changed, will need to have blood-donor tubing available.
		Effective wound drainage system supports healing.
		
		Documentation of drain output q shift.

• Lymphedema	1. No pillow under affected arm, except at night, because it discourages movement (unless specifically ordered by physician).
	2. Exercises:
	  a. Start with extension-flexion of fingers, supination-pronation of forearm, ADL.
	  b. Check with physician regarding abduction and shoulder movement.
	3. Reach to Recovery program: Check with surgeon regarding permission and exercise restrictions. Fill out referral form and call American Cancer Society. Keep form on front of chart.
	4. No BP or blood to be drawn from arm on affected side.
	  a. Mark Kardex accordingly.
	  b. Specify on requisitions.
	  c. Inform patient.
	  d. Sign over bed with information.
		By fifth POD: Patient performing ADLs with affected arm.
		
		Documentation of patient's progress in performing ADLs with affected arm.
		
		Referral form completed and sent to appropriate agency.
		
		Patient can explain reasons for protecting arm on affected side.

Continued on next page.

FIGURE 4-3 continued

Potential problems	Nursing intervention or management	Outcome

• Wound infection	1. After original dressing removed by physician:
	  a. Check incision for redness, swelling, drainage, separation, increased tenderness.
	  b. Check temperature as stated above.
	2. Wound care.
	  a. Change dressings prn (at least qd).
	  b. Use sterile technique.
	  c. Assess type and amount of drainage.
	  d. Use minimal tape near incision and remove carefully.
	  e. Keep incision dry. Patient may shower 24 hours after drains are removed. Pat incision dry and apply 4 x 4 over drain sites if drainage still present.
		Within 48 hours prior to discharge:
		Patient afebrile. Exceptions: Physician notified.
		From clinical record, evidence that temp < 99.6°.
		Incision clean and intact at time of discharge.

• Accumulation of fluid	1. Check for puffiness or swelling under skin flaps, both while tubes are in and after they are removed. 2. Evaluate patient's C/O fullness and increased tenderness. Notify physician if occurs. Aspiration may be necessary.	
• Change of body image	1. Assess patient's previous body image and family relationships. Plan intervention accordingly. 2. Minimize embarrassment. Cover drainage bottle with bag. 3. Involve patient in incisional care. 4. Nurse should be with patient when she views incision for first time. Initial viewing should be based on patient's readiness but should be sometime prior to discharge. 5. Reach to Recovery supplies temporary prosthesis. Explanation instructions listed below. Patient should have similar list to take home.	Patient shows some degree of acceptance of surgical outcome. Progress notes from third POD to discharge show that patient verbalizes acceptance, or patient is able to look at incision, asking questions regarding home care. Patient verbalizes understanding of discharge instructions and given teaching plan. Progress notes must show that patient understands instructions.

- Recurrence of disease

1. Teach patient how to monitor self-care.
   Activity. No heavy lifting or straining. Activity as tolerated. Take rest periods at intervals. May do light housekeeping, activities of daily living, use stairs, maintain program of arm exercises as ordered by physician. Check with physician regarding resumption of sports and driving.
   Arm care. Avoid injections, blood pressures, or venipunctures in affected arm. Avoid sunburn. Be careful when cooking to prevent burning hand; guard against scratches, insect bites, hangnails on affected side. See physician for breaks in skin and swelling of arm.
   Incisional care. May shower, pat dry over incision. Keep area clean and dry. Observe for any type of drainage and increased tenderness in area.
   Breast self-exam. Do breast self-examination monthly seven to 10 days after period (if after menopause, at the same time each month). Report any change, lump, or thickening to physician.
2. Teach BSE.

Patient knows follow-up care measures.

Patient able to demonstrate correct technique for BSE.

PATIENT INSTRUCTION: BREAST SELF-EXAMINATION

The BSE has two parts, inspection and palpation.

Inspection. Sit or stand in front of a mirror. Inspect your breasts with your arms at your sides and raised above your head and while contracting your chest muscles.

Note breast size, symmetry, shape, and the direction the nipples are pointing (inverted or normal). Compare what your breasts look like when you change arm positions. Look for dimpling, puckering; note skin changes, swelling, red patches, orange-like texture.

Palpation. While lying on your back, squeeze each nipple to see if there is a discharge (discharge does not necessarily mean cancer).

Palpate each breast, using the pads of the first three fingers of your hand opposite the breast. In examining your left breast, for example, place your left hand behind your head and examine with your right hand. Move your hand in a circular motion, beginning near the nipple, making gradually larger circles. Palpate into the underarm area and above the collar bone.

All breast tissue is somewhat lumpy. Tumors are usually hard, irregular in shape, and appear more often in the upper outer section of the breast.

● *Modified radical mastectomy:* Removal of all
   breast tissue and part or all of the pectoralis
   minor and axillary nodes. The pectoral
   muscles are kept intact. In recent years, the
   modified radical mastectomy has become
   widely used because studies have shown that
   the survival rate is about the same as that
   with more radical procedures.

Perioperative   ● A drain (Hemovac, Vacutainer bottle, test-
notes: tube) that creates a means of suction
                       (vacuum) is often inserted during surgery to
                       collect fluid away from the operative site to
                       decrease swelling, limit discoloration, and
                       promote healing.

Special postoperative care and teaching

Psychological support

Emotional support is of paramount importance to the woman—usually
30–60 years of age—who has just undergone gross disfigurement of her
body through a mastectomy. Not only does she have concerns about
long-term survival, but she needs assistance in coping with the multiple
implications of the surgery, ranging from her relationship with her
spouse to proper fit of her clothing.

Some hospitals arrange for mastectomy support groups. At Evanston
Hospital, recent mastectomy patients meet once a week with an RN
to discuss the various aspects of their postoperative readjustment. Breast
reconstruction procedures performed either at the time of mastectomy
or several months later reduce the trauma of disfigurement associated
with mastectomy.

The American Cancer Society also provides a mastectomy volunteer
visiting service. Mastectomy patients can be referred to this service.
An effective way to initiate referral is through a permission form completed in cooperation with the physician (Figure 4-4). After the referral
form is filled out, the nurse calls the volunteer visiting service and
provides information about the patient, including family history—
spouse, friend, or responsible person, and number of children—and, if
the patient will require a breast prosthesis, the patient's preoperative
bra size. A volunteer visit is scheduled prior to the patient's discharge
from the hospital. If possible, family members are included in the visit.

Mastectomy Exercises

Several exercises have been developed to aid the patient to regain full
range of motion and use of the affected side and arm. Exercises are

FIGURE 4-4 MASTECTOMY VOLUNTEER VISITING SERVICE

Patient's name _____ Date _____

Room number _____

DOCTOR'S ORDER:

PLEASE VISIT THIS PATIENT   _____

Demonstrate simple exercise   _____

Omit exercise   _____

Indicate date for visit   _____

                                           Physician

Remarks:

— —

(To be filled out by nurse)

Patient's name _____ Age _____ Room no. _____

Address _____ Phone _____

Marital status _____ Husband's name _____

Children (ages and sex) __ _____

Surgeon _____

Date of surgery _____ Side of surgery _____ Bra size _____

Approximate date of discharge _____

                               _____ R.N.

Remarks:

usually begun by the fourth or fifth postoperative day. Teach your patient through explanation and demonstration how to perform the exercises. Patients require appropriate pain control, reinforcement, and
support to perform and repeat the routines several times each day. Exercises should not be painful. Emphasize bilateral activity and good
posture. Inform patient that it takes weeks for stiffness and heaviness
to go away.

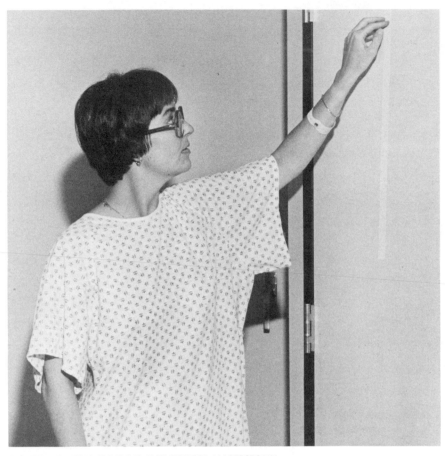

FIGURE 4-5. WALL-CLIMBING EXERCISE FOR MASTECTOMY
PATIENT. RECORD OF PROGRESS IS KEPT BY MARKING ON
TAPE THE HEIGHT PATIENT CAN REACH.

Even during the first 24 hours postoperatively, the patient should
begin to perform certain activities of daily living (ADL) that involve
arm movement. Encourage hair brushing, eating, and similar activities
with affected arm.

Wall-climbing exercises should be started to enable the patient
eventually to raise both arms straight up, close to the head. *Position:*
Hands comfortably close to and facing the wall, with feet apart. *Instructions:* Have the hand crawl up the wall above the head. Before
starting the next climb, hand should be lowered to shoulder level.
Progress in each reach is noted by marking the height attained on tape
placed on the wall (Figure 4-5).

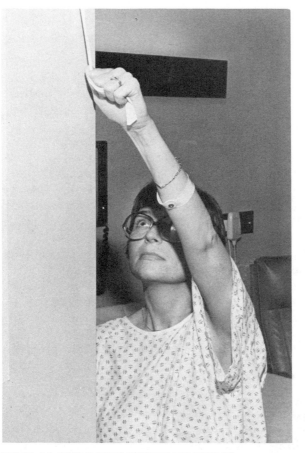

FIGURE 4-6. ROPE-PULLING EXERCISE FOR POST-OP
MASTECTOMY PATIENT.

Rope exercise: Tie one end of a rope onto doorknob. *Position:* Stand alongside the rope and at a right angle to the door, looking straight ahead. *Instructions:* Start making small circles with the rope, moving the entire arm from the shoulder. Eventually make larger circles, moving closer to the door. Exercise should be done at first five times in one direction and five times in the other.

Rope pulling exercises: Throw a rope over the door. *Position:* Stand or sit facing edge of door with feet on either side of the door (Figure 4-6). *Instructions:* Pull down on rope with the unaffected arm; this will cause you to raise the affected arm. Start five times twice each day and increase as much as can be tolerated.

The following are other exercises the patient should learn. They ought to be performed in front of a mirror so that patient can check for proper posture.

1. To strengthen the muscles in the hand and forearm, make a fist with the unaffected side and squeeze it with the other hand, then release the fist and repeat several times. This exercise will also help increase circulation in the arm.
2. Sitting or standing, hold cane or umbrella, hands spread apart approximately shoulder width, with right hand under, left hand on top. Put right hand at left hip and, with right hand leading, lift cane up over right shoulder, cane pointing to ceiling. Return cane to starting position. Head and eyes follow right hand. *Switch hands,* lift up over left shoulder. This will help increase range of motion of the shoulders.
3. Sitting or standing, hold cane or umbrella, hands spread apart approximately shoulder width, with both hands on top. Start with arms straight down in front of your hips. Keeping arms straight, lift cane up in front of you, stopping when hands are just above your head. Return cane to starting position. Don't lean backward while performing this exercise.
4. Sitting or lying on back, clasp fingers behind neck. Bring elbows together in front of your face; then spread elbows as far apart as possible. This will help to improve your posture.
5. One hand behind head, the other behind low back, grasp towel with both hands. Hand on side of the mastectomy holds towel behind low back. Pull towel up and down as if you were drying your back. This exercise will help you to clasp your bra behind your back.

Precautions

Injections, venipunctures, or blood pressures must not be taken on the patient's affected arm. A reminder sign should be placed above the patient's bed to warn hospital staff of these precautions, and the patient should be informed about the need to avoid using the affected arm for these procedures.

Following hospitalization, the patient should take care to avoid injury to the affected arm when performing activities of daily living such as cooking. Teach her hand precautions to help avoid infections. Here is a guide to teaching about hand precautions:

Hand Precautions

After a radical or modified radical mastectomy, your arm may swell because lymph nodes and vessels were removed, and your body is less able to combat infection in this arm. The following is a brief summary of precautions you can take to help prevent infection and swelling of the arm.

To help prevent infection

- Avoid having vaccinations, injections, blood drawing on your affected arm. If necessary, remind medical and nursing people to use the opposite arm.
- To avoid burns when cooking, use a mitt to cover your hand and arm while you are at the stove.
- Instead of cutting hangnails, use lanolin-based cream to keep your cuticles soft.
- Take care of cuts and scrapes promptly by washing with soap and using an antiseptic.
- When you garden, wear heavy gloves. When you sew, use a thimble. When you are cleaning with steel wool, wear rubber gloves. Whatever you're doing, avoid puncturing the skin.
- If you smoke, light matches and hold your cigarette with the unaffected hand.
- Wait to shave or apply deodorant under the affected arm until your doctor has given you permission. Until the surgical wound is healed, chemicals in the deodorant may irritate the incision. Take extra care when you are allowed to shave, since this area may be numb. This is due to nerves being cut during the surgery. Some numbness may persist for months.

Contact your doctor if any signs of infection occur in your arm—redness, increased warmth, hardness, or swelling.

To help prevent swelling

- Ask for help when lifting anything heavy, especially the first few weeks after surgery when the incision is still healing or swelling is present.
- Carry your purse on the unaffected arm to avoid pressure or heavy weight on your weaker arm.
- Avoid clothing and jewelry that constrict your affected operative arm—tight watches, elasticized apparel. Carrying heavy objects or wearing constricting clothes may decrease the circulation in your arm and thereby cause swelling.
- If you want to tan yourself, expose this area to the sun gradually to prevent burning. If you have to be exposed to the sun for a long time, cover your affected side. Two lotions that are effective are Sun Eclipse—regular or total—and Pre-Sun #8 or #15. Both contain sunscreen.

COLON, RECTUM (Figure 4-7—see page 92)

Procedures:
- *Hemicolectomy:* Removal of one-half of the colon.
- *Left hemicolectomy:* Removal of colon from the middle of the transverse segment to the rectum.
- *Right hemicolectomy:* Removal of colon from the ileum to the middle of the transverse segment.
- *Colectomy:* Removal of part or all of the colon. For example, a posterior colectomy involves removal of the lower portion of the colon and may include the rectum.
- *Sigmoid resection:* Removal of part or all of the sigmoid colon.
- *Anterior/low anterior resection:* Anterior approach to lesions of lower colon. Primary anastomoses are accomplished when possible.
- *Abdominal-perineal resection:* Removal of rectum, usually through both a perineal and an abdominal incision with a permanent colostomy. The trend is to leave the perineal incision open, allowing for secondary closure.

Preoperative care

To facilitate visibility and ease of surgery and to prevent contamination of the peritoneal cavity during the operation, most surgeons prescribe preoperative cleansing of the bowel. There are several regimens for bowel preparation. Common elements include:

- a clear liquid diet and multiple enemas for two to three days pre-operatively and
- prophylactic neomycin and erythromycin to prevent postoperative wound infections.

In some cases, the patient may be started on systemic antibiotics the day before surgery.

A colostomy may be temporary or permanent. Whichever it is, a colostomy results in drastic alteration of body image, and the primary nurse plays a key role in aiding the patient's emotional as well as practical adjustment to it.

Temporary colostomy. Performed to either relieve an obstruction or as part of a two-stage operative approach to removal of the lesion. In the two-stage approach, the colostomy may be permanent, depending on the findings at the time of surgery and the extent of bowel removed. The first-stage operation is done to construct the colostomy. In the second-stage operation, the colostomy is either closed (take down) or a permanent colostomy is constructed.

Permanent colostomy. Performed to provide an external opening for expulsion of feces.

The level of the bowel resection determines the method of postoperative bowel control. Before surgery, the stoma site is marked to ensure that the colostomy orifice will be appropriate to the patient's body build and clothing. Be sure that the patient is informed of the procedure and its effects before surgery; provide initial information about postoperative management and the postoperative resources that are planned to assist the patient to learn to manage bowel function. Teaching should be planned to accommodate the patient's level of understanding and anxiety.

Perioperative care

During colorectal surgery, the surgeon may resect the tumor and perform an end-to-end anastomosis. Alternatively, the surgeon may elect to perform a colostomy.

When a colostomy is necessary, a stoma is constructed by suturing part of the bowel to the abdominal wall or bringing the bowel to the surface through a separation of the muscle. There are three major types of colostomies:

Transverse loop colostomy. To form a transverse loop colostomy, a loop of the bowel is brought to the abdominal surface, and a transverse incision is made to drain fecal contents. The loop is secured in place temporarily with a plastic bridge or rod, usually for five to six days postoperatively. In many cases, the transverse loop colostomy is a temporary measure. The fecal contents will be liquid, and regulation of bowel function through daily irrigations will not be feasible.

Double-barrel colostomy. A double-barrel colostomy is constructed by bringing the proximal and distal portions of the bowel to the surface. The proximal loop requires an ostomy appliance to collect fecal contents. Initially, the distal loop will have a watery, mucoid discharge that eventually ceases. Don't be alarmed if fecal contents are excreted via the rectum. This excretion occurs with inadequate bowel cleansing prior to the operation and lasts only for a few days.

Involvement of the sigmoid colon: When the sigmoid, or descending colon is involved in the resection, the surgeon will attempt to leave the splenic flexure intact to enable some form of bowel control later. The necessary margins are resected, and the distal portion may either be sutured closed, or a mucus fistula is constructed.

Continued on page 96.

FIGURE 4-7 NURSING THE COLOSTOMY OR ILEOSTOMY PATIENT

Potential problems	Nursing intervention or management	Outcome
• Circulatory impairment or bleeding	**Immediate post-op ostomy care** Check stoma during first 24- 48-hour period for: a. Color—expect bright red appearance of stoma. b. Drainage—small amount of serosanguineous. c. Skin condition. d. Vaseline gauze around stoma. e. Size of stoma, retracted or protracted.	Viable stoma, no bleeding.
• Skin breakdown from: a. acid and enzymes present in stomal drainage b. irritation from bag	Within 24 hours, unless ordered otherwise, place ostomy bag over stoma as follows: a. Measure size of stoma and order appropriate bags from central supply. Assemble equipment. b. Wash around stoma, removing surgical prep, using soap and water, rinse *well*, pat dry. c. Prepare stoma appliance as per manufacturer's instructions. Take care that appliance fits snugly around stoma. d. Do not put holes in bag until peristalsis and drainage is established. e. Do not change bag in A.M. until physician has opportunity to evaluate type and amount of drainage for the first few post-op days. NOTE: One type of appliance, the Karaya Seal Ring, contains the gum Karaya. The Karaya Seal Ring may vary widely in color and is affected by changes in temperature and humidity. Indoor air is generally drier in the winter, tending to make the Karaya Seal feel firmer and less tacky. Before applying, simply moisten the Karaya Seal with a touch of warm water. This will provide a proper surface for satisfactory adhesion.	Skin integrity maintained around stoma. Patient able to perform colostomy self-care and fit appliance properly. Return of bowel function by third to fourth POD.

• Skin breakdown around stoma

Routine skin care daily and prn
1. Eliminate cause of any skin irritation if possible.
2. Cleanse area with water. Use soap only if absolutely necessary and then rinse well, pat dry.
3. If irritation is deep and looks moist, a heat lamp may be used. Place lamp with 75- or 100-watt bulb over area, 12 inches away, for 10 minutes. Keep moist 4 x 4 over stoma while light is on.
4. If necessary, apply light coat of Amphoel over area and dry until chalky.
5. If working on colostomy or open wound, protect the opening and spray Amphoel area with Rezifilm.
6. If special skin problem arises, stoma adhesive can be applied around stoma. Cut to fit stoma as well as possible. Apply bag over this.
7. Use appropriate preparations to protect macerated skin. Then apply bag.

Routine bag changes daily and prn
Some patients with a well-fitting seal and no skin problems who have a drainable stoma bag may not need to change bag daily, but bag should be drained daily and prn and rinsed from bottom with syringe filled with water, and a deodorant should be inserted.

Irrigation of ostomies
1. Ileostomies are never irrigated unless obstructed. Done by physician.
2. In double-barrel colostomies, the proximal (active) stoma is usually the one irrigated. Check with physician to be sure which is the proximal stoma and which is the distal.

Prevention or earliest possible resolution of skin problem.

Patient has adequate drainage, is comfortable and odor-free as possible.

Continued on next page.

FIGURE 4-7 continued

Potential problems	Nursing intervention or management	Outcome
• Complications at home secondary to inadequate teaching of colostomy irrigation	Teach patient colostomy irrigation procedure (see below) and related dietary-control measures	Control of colon mastered by patient or significant others prior to discharge.

COLOSTOMY IRRIGATION PROCEDURE

1. Assemble equipment.
   a. Irrigation bag. If not available, use enema bag with nipple from baby bottle.
   b. Finger cot with lubricating jelly.
   c. Waxed bag, Handi Wipes, or toilet paper and bath towel.
   d. Elastic belt and drainage bag.
2. Obtain specific order from physician about irrigation procedure.
   a. Type of solution
   b. Amount of irrigation—usually 250 cc for first irrigation procedure, gradually increasing in increments of 250 cc until total of 1000 cc, if tolerated.
3. Prepare patient.
   a. Use calm, unhurried manner.
   b. Explain all steps of procedure and reasons to patient.

h. Lubricate tip of irrigation tube and gently insert into stoma. Never force a tube. If a resistance is felt, stop at that position and allow the water to flow. Gradually insert the remaining tubing until you reach four inches. Hold disc firm against stoma to prevent loss of water.

i. Allow five to 10 minutes for 250–500 cc to run in and 10–15 minutes for 500–1000 cc. If cramping occurs, stop water flow and wait until cramp subsides before continuing with remaining amount.

j. Remove tube and clean off with tissue. Allow 30–45 minutes for evacuation. A gentle abdominal massage will stimulate evacuation.

k. Clamp irrigation bag at bottom if patient desires. He may ambulate or do other hygiene care during this period.

l. Record results—amount and consistency of irrigation return—on chart. If no return on initial irrigation, don't panic.

c. Discuss with patient his anticipated schedule at home and try whenever possible to correlate hospital irrigation time with when patient will do it at home.

d. If patient has long-standing colostomy, try to follow patient's own schedule and technique.

4. Irrigation technique:

a. Prepare prescribed amount of solution, usually tepid tap water.

b. Flush tube to remove air bubbles.

c. If Hollister bag is used, slide disc to #4. Hang water bag in front of patient and at level to allow bottom of bag to hang between patient's ear and shoulder (no more than 18" above stoma). Moisten sponge disc on irrigation drain.

d. Position patient on commode and drape with bath towel.

1) If A/P was done, patient may sit on chair in front of commode and use "donut" for comfort.

2) A pillow may be placed at patient's back for comfort when he is sitting on commode.

e. Remove colostomy pouch and clean area as much as possible with toilet tissue or Handi Wipes.

f. Dilate stoma if prescribed. Check for tightness of stoma and direction of colon.

g. Attach irrigation drain to colostomy belt and allow end of drain to drop into commode.

Wait until next day and irrigate again. Reasons for no return include:

1) Dehydration (good idea to drink a glass of water prior to irrigation).

2) Insufficient amount of fluid.

3) Catheter inserted too far.

If on the second day you still have no results, notify physician.

m. When completed, wash skin and dry well. If skin is irritated, do skin care.

n. Apply colostomy bag.

o. If patient's condition is stable, sutures are out, and physician orders it, patient may shower or take tub bath.

5. If patient is unable to tolerate bathroom irrigation, drain irrigation bag into bedpan with patient positioned on side.

Postoperative care and teaching

Colostomy care begins before surgery with selection of a stoma site and preoperative teaching. Following surgery, there are several major elements to be included in the patient's care:

1. *Selection of a properly fitting appliance.* Initially, the patient may require a larger size because of postoperative edema of the stoma. As the swelling recedes, the patient should be fitted with an appliance that fits snugly over, but does not constrict, the stoma. The type of appliance and length of the collection bag depend on the patient's body build and location of the stoma. A wide variety of ostomy products are available, and the primary nurse in consultation with an enterostomal therapist should guide and aid the patient in becoming knowledgeable and comfortable in the application and use of these products. Time and patience are necessary in the successful teaching of a patient and family on colostomy self-care. Frequently, the patient may feel that this is a distasteful responsibility to assume, and well-planned nursing care in the readjustment process can help the patient overcome aversion to it.

2. Colostomy irrigations are like a daily enema and in many cases may enable the patient to have control of bowel function, particularly following a sigmoid resection. When teaching colostomy irrigation, consider the patient's sensitivities. You can support the patient with a calm approach when assisting him or her to accept these irrigations as a daily routine. A well-thought-out step-by-step teaching plan is essential. Eventually, as regular bowel function is established, the patient may not need to wear an appliance or may choose to wear a closed bag or pouch.

3. Odor control is an important part of the ostomy patient's personal hygiene. There are several types of ostomy deodorants available. Also, the patient should be instructed to limit or avoid foods that may produce odor or flatulence.

4. Care of the skin surrounding the stoma begins the first day after surgery. It is important to keep the area surrounding the stoma clean. Proper application of the appliance is essential. The skin should be correctly prepared, and a good seal obtained, to avoid wrinkles and skin folds, thus preventing leakage of fecal contents onto the surrounding skin (Figures 4-8 to 4-12).

5. The frequency of bag changes should be kept to a minimum to avoid skin irritation and breakdown. The bag or pouch should be cleansed daily and emptied of its contents on a regular basis.

6. Signs of infection, rash, or skin breakdown should be noted, and, when they occur, immediate corrective action should be taken. The physician should be notified.

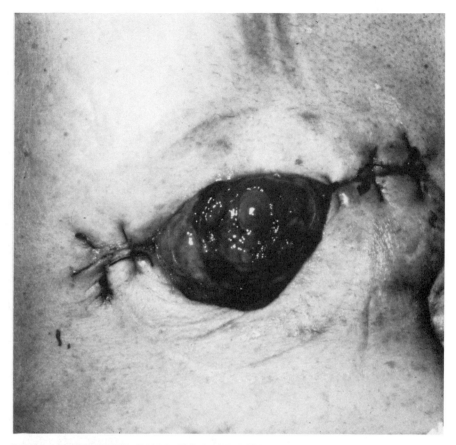

FIGURE 4-8. AREA OF SKIN THAT SURROUNDS THE STOMA
SITE MUST BE KEPT CLEAN.

Summary

Always remember that in the early postoperative days the patient receives both verbal and nonverbal messages from his care givers. The primary nurse must maintain a mature, competent approach to successfully help the patient adjust to the colostomy and incorporate this change into his or her altered body image. Sensing that you approach the colostomy with displeasure tends to reinforce negative feelings that may delay the patient's acceptance process.

Wound care. Wound irrigations are required for patients who have had a perineal resection without primary closure. Irrigations are usually ordered three to four times each day to keep the area clean and avoid infection.

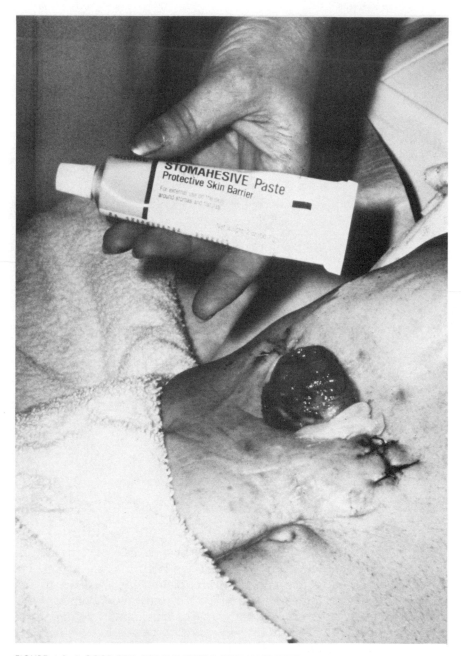

FIGURE 4-9. A GOOD SEAL FOR THE STOMA APPLIANCE KEEPS
FECAL MATERIAL FROM THE SURROUNDING SKIN.

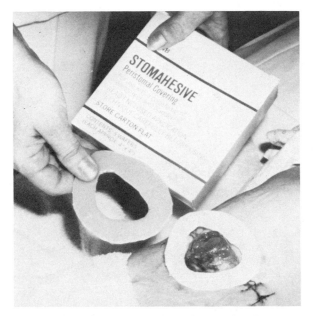

FIGURE 4-10. A PERISTOMAL COVERING IS PLACED ON THE
SEAL FOR THE APPLIANCE.

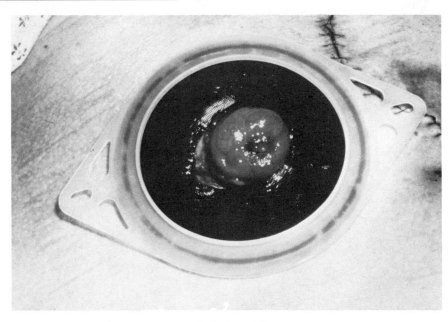

FIGURE 4-11. THE COLOSTOMY APPLIANCE SHOULD FIT
SNUGLY OVER THE STOMA.

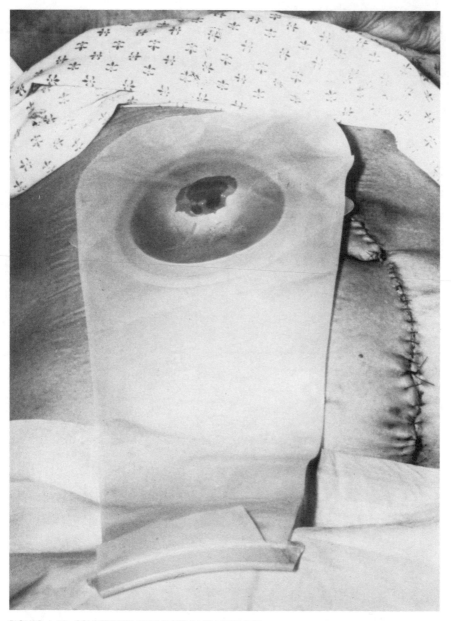

FIGURE 4-12. COLOSTOMY APPLIANCE IN PLACE WITH
COLLECTION BAG ATTACHED.

Rectal packing with secondary closure is utilized for some patients to control excessive bleeding. Ideally, the packing should be in one piece to avoid leaving any material within the wound, which would be a potential source of infection. You need to monitor the area regularly, using a good light source, to observe the healing process.

Insertion of surgical drains may be done for patients with primary closure. These drains are connected to suction for several days postoperatively. Surgeon preference dictates which approach is selected.

LUNG (Figures 4-13—see page 102—and 4-14—see page 104)

Procedure:	• **Thoracotomy:** Excision of a lung tumor. • **Pneumonectomy:** Removal of the lung.
Preoperative:	Patients undergo an extensive diagnostic workup before surgery, including cytology examination of sputum, pulmonary function screening, and possible bronchoscopy.
Perioperative:	A lateral incision, either posterior or anterior, is the most commonly used approach. A chest tube is inserted at the time of surgery to promote lung re-expansion and fluid drainage.

Postoperative nursing care

1. The patient may be cared for in the intensive care unit during the initial 24–48 hour postoperative period and should be prepared before surgery, possibly with a tour of the unit.
2. You must understand how chest tubes and water-seal drainage function. During the thoracotomy procedure, air enters the pleural space, disrupting its normal negative pressure state. Therefore, chest tubes are inserted to allow for the removal of air and to prevent accumulation of secretions. The chest tube is then connected to a water-seal drainage system and may or may not be connected to a suction source. There are various types of drainage systems available. The chest tube remains in place for several days and is observed for possible development of an air leak. If an air leak occurs, the doctor is immediately notified.
3. A major goal of the postoperative course for the thoracotomy patient is to regain or restore either the previous or an improved level of respiratory function. You must be especially diligent in encouraging breathing exercises, coughing, use of incentive spirometry and active ambulation.

FIGURE 4-13 TEACHING THE PRE-OP THORACOTOMY PATIENT

Learning needs	Patient education	Evaluation
• Simple explanation of anatomy and physiology of respiratory system	1. Show diagram of chest to patient to facilitate explanation. 2. See below for basic physiology.	Patient able to state anatomy and physiology in own words. ☐ Yes ☐ No
• Simple explanation to patient and/or significant other about the disease process, the purpose of the operation, and procedure itself	1. Reinforce physician's explanation of purpose of operation. 2. Explain type of incision. 3. Reinforce physician's explanation. Allow patients to ask questions. Refer to physician if there are any serious reservations or misunderstandings on part of patient.	Patient and/or significant other understands purpose and procedure through physician's explanation and reinforcement by nurse. Patient psychologically prepared for surgery. ☐ Yes ☐ No

• Explanation of chest tubes to patients with wedge resection or lobectomy (usually don't use after pneumonectomy)	1. Physical characteristics of chest tube: size, diameter, length.
	2. Purpose and placement (see below and again use diagram of chest to explain tube placement).
	3. Anchored by sutures. Skin seals to prevent leakage.
	4. Demonstrate with sample tubes if they are available.
	5. Chest tubes should remain coiled on bed and below level of chest; Pleur-evac kept upright.
	6. Chest tubes left in as long as necessary (usually two to five days) until:
	  a. No air leak.
	  b. Lung re-expanded.
	  c. Fluid drainage minimal.
		Patient able to verbalize implications of chest tube.
		☐ Yes ☐ No

• Explanation of rationale for coughing and deep breathing	1. Increased mucous secretions from anesthesia. 2. Demonstrate coughing and deep breathing to promote full lung expansion. Explain splinting and availability of meds to control pain.	Patient able to demonstrate coughing and deep breathing and importance of these. ☐ Yes ☐ No

Patient can demonstrate use of incentive spirometer if ordered.
[ ] Yes [ ] No

Patient able to verbalize importance of post-op activity even with chest tube.
[ ] Yes [ ] No

3. Explain and demonstrate incentive spirometer, if ordered.

• Special considerations

1. Teach special post-op routines of recovery room and ICU.
2. pHisohex or soap-and-water shower evening before operation, as ordered (also just before surgery if time allows).
3. Explain hazards of smoking.
4. Teach importance of sitting and ambulating after operation.
5. Encourage use of arm on affected side for ADL for optimum return of muscle tonicity.
6. Thoracotomy pull rope facilitates activity.
7. A nurse from ICU may do pre-op visit.
8. Physical therapist may visit for breathing exercises and/or chest percussion, if ordered by physician.

RESPIRATORY SYSTEM: Primary purpose is to take in O_2 and give off CO_2.

1. Organs
   a. Nose
   b. Mouth and pharynx
   c. Larynx (throat)
   d. Trachea (windpipe) and tracheal branches (bronchi and bronchioles)
   e. Lung tissue into which small extensions of the bronchi reach
2. Anatomy & Physiology—basically, lungs act as bellows: inhale, air in; exhale, waste out.
   a. Lungs are separated by trachea, on right three lobes, on left two lobes.
   b. Lungs protected by ribs and skin of outer chest wall.
   c. Both lungs enclosed in moist membrane called pleura.
   d. Chest wall has similar lining.
   e. When air taken in and lungs expand, the two pleura come very close together. Because they are moistened with special fluid, they do not cause friction and pain when you breathe. The space is called pleural cavity.
   f. Whenever the chest is entered surgically (or traumatically) air and fluid settle into the space between the pleura. This causes the lung on that side to collapse.
   g. Effective breathing is compromised when the lungs are collapsed. For this reason, air and fluid in the pleural space must be gotten rid of.
   h. This is done by the insertion of a chest tube into the pleural space. The chest tube is placed into the region where it will most fully do its job, then attached to an apparatus or receptacle for air and fluid to escape.
   i. When the lung is re-expanded, the chest tube can be removed, and the process of respiration can proceed naturally, as before.

FIGURE 4-14 NURSING THE THORACOTOMY PATIENT

Potential problems	Nursing intervention or management	Outcome

• Respiratory failure	1. BP, P, R q1-2h for first 24 hours. Temp q4h. May take more frequently or for longer time if evidence of hypoxia:
	  a. cyanosis
	  b. confusion
	  c. restlessness
	  d. rapid, shallow respirations
	  e. tachycardia
	  f. hypertension or hypotension
	2. O_2 therapy as ordered:
	  a. O_2 per nasal prongs @ 2–5/min. most commonly ordered.
	  b. if aerosol face mask or high humidity face tent ordered, patient must use nasal prongs when eating.
	  c. Assess need for portable O_2 during transfer from ICU.
	3. Blood gases as ordered or as indicated by respiratory condition.
	4. Head of bed raised to 45° or more, or patient in chair. Armchair with broad back preferred.
	5. After chest tube removed, continue to observe for respiratory distress and cough and deep breathe patient. If respiratory treatment previously ordered, review need for continuation after chest tube is removed.
		ICU discharge status
		The patient will not require O_2 therapy.
		Exceptions:
		  a. Previous COPD or other pre-existing chronic respiratory or vascular condition.
		  b. Nursing assessment that there is a clinical need for O_2, either continuously or for the transfer to the floor.
		Documentation that the patient was not S.O.B. with activity, that respirations were easy and unlabored, and/or that the respiratory rate was less than 16–20/minute.

• Inadequate expansion of lungs due to malfunction of the chest tubes	Monitor chest tube systems (see below) for proper functioning q1-2h for first 24 hours and as indicated thereafter.	Properly functioning chest tube. Documentation of the development of an air leak and any corrective measures instituted.

PROCEDURE FOR MONITORING CHEST TUBES

Chest tubes should be checked for the following:

a. Patency.

b. Fluctuation of fluid in chambers with respirations.

c. Amount and types of drainage; record q shift or more frequently if indicated. If chest tube output > 100 cc/hr, notify service stat.

d. Air-tight connection of all tubing.

e. Integrity of plastic Pleur-evac.

f. Emerson suction pump as ordered.

g. Keep Pleur-evac upright and below level of waist.

h. Keep tubing unkinked and coiled on bed to avoid dependent loops.

i. Lift tubes to drain q2h, rather than milking them; do not allow backflow toward chest.

j. Maintain desired level of solution in suction control chamber and water seal chamber by adding sterile solution through openings prn.

k. For further information, refer to manual for purposes and care of Pleur-evac and/or chest bottle drainage system.

● Interruptions in closed chest drainage system

1. If tube dislodges from chest, apply pressure dressing stat and notify service. Notify X-ray of necessity of stat chest films.

2. Possible emergency situations and appropriate nursing management:

   a. Pleur-evac cracks or collection chambers are full: Call service to change. Chest X-ray will probably be ordered.

   b. Tubes become disconnected: Reconnect and call service. Chest X-ray will probably be ordered.

   c. Air leak anywhere in system (as evidenced by persistent bubbling in the water seal chamber): Never clamp; call service.

   d. Clogged tubes: Call service.

   e. In general, chest tubes should never be clamped except for brief interval while Pleur-evac is being changed.

3. Removal of tube requires the following equipment: dressing pack, Vaseline gauze, 4 x 4's, 3" waterproof tape, bath towel.

Effective chest drainage; maximum lung expansion.

Documentation of the development of any air leak and of corrective measures instituted.

Documentation of removal of chest tubes, appearance of site, and type of dressing applied.

Continued on next page.

FIGURE 4-14 continued

Potential problems	Nursing intervention or management	Outcome

• Atelectasis and/or pneumonia	1. Cough and deep breathe at least qh or as indicated by amount of secretion.
	2. Suction prn. If pneumonectomy, check with physician before suctioning.
	3. Auscultate chest for breath sounds as indicated.
	4. Use incentive spirometer as ordered.
	5. Turn to back and either side at least q2h. Pull rope to assist patient with activity.
	6. Implement early mobility. Pneumonectomy patients must not be turned with operated side up for several weeks. Mobility of patient slower with pneumonectomy. Ambulation usually begins within first 24 hours.
	7. Temp q4h, more often if indicated.
	8. Protocol for post-op chest X-rays:
	  a. Usually order upright, PA portable films.
	  b. If patient sent to X-ray, nurse should:
	    1) Check about need for portable O₂.
	    2) Take precautions against excessive patient waits in department.
		Documentation of breath sounds.
		
		By time of discharge
		1. Lungs clear as demonstrated by clinical signs.
		Exception: Previous COPD or other pre-existing chronic respiratory or vascular condition. Following must be documented in progress notes within 48 hours before discharge:
		  Temp < 99.6°
		  No productive cough
		  Deep breathes easily
		2. Ambulating length of hall without dyspnea.
		Exception: Previous existing incapacity to ambulate. Ambulation must be documented in progress notes within 72 hours prior to discharge.

• Shoulder immobility

Encourage ADL with both arms, especially arm on affected side.

• Incisional problems

1. Observe for signs of incisional infection and report accordingly.
2. Apply Betadine ointment to chest tube insertion site bid.
3. Reassure patient that swelling in upper part of incision is expected (especially with posterolateral incision).
4. Day after chest tubes are removed, remove dressing and allow tub bath or shower.

• Respiratory infections

Patient should:
1. Discourage visitors with colds or illness.
2. Avoid large crowds.
3. Know necessity of surgical follow-up. Make sure patient knows day of doctor's appointment.
4. Take medications only as directed.
5. Check with doctor regarding resumption of physical labor and vigorous sports.
6. Not drive until surgeon allows.
7. Check with physician about flu shot, especially in the fall.
8. Follow physician's instructions regarding baths and showers, stairs.

Documentation that patient or significant other able to list instructions for home care.

THYROID (Figure 4-15—see page 110)

Procedure:	• *Total thyroidectomy:* Resection of the entire thyroid gland.
	• *Subtotal thyroidectomy:* Removal of one-half or more of the gland.
	• *Lobectomy:* Removal of one lobe of the thyroid gland.
Perioperative:	Care is taken to identify and preserve the parathyroid glands.

Postoperative nursing care
Points in postoperative care to be emphasized are as follows:

- A tracheostomy set is kept at the bedside in the event of respiratory distress.
- For the initial 24-hour period, closely monitor the calcium levels and watch for signs of hypocalcemia.
- To avoid tension on the suture line, the patient is not to cough.

Post-thyroidectomy patient instructions
1. You have had a (total-subtotal) thyroidectomy and must take a thyroid preparation the rest of your life.
2. You are on _____ (milligrams-grains) of thyroid every _____ . Your doctor will prescribe the specific replacement therapy for diminished or absent thyroid function.

Side effects of thyroid medication may occur as your body needs for thyroid change. These side effects may include:

- sweating,
- heart palpitations with or without pain,
- weight loss,
- diarrhea, and
- nervousness.

Notify your doctor if any of these symptoms occur so that he can adjust the dosage of thyroid to your needs.

3. If your doctor has prescribed oral calcium supplements, make sure you understand the dosage and length of treatment.

Calcium is essential for many body functions, and calcium requirements change over time. Symptoms of low calcium may include:

- irritability,
- tingling around the lips,

- muscle twitching,
- cramping in legs or abdomen,
- numbness or tingling in extremities, and
- sometimes nausea and vomiting.

Notify your doctor if these symptoms occur, as your calcium medication may need to be increased.

Check with your doctor as to when you may resume the following activities:

Driving car_____   Lifting_____
Returning to work _ _____   Singing (or public speaking) _____
Diet_____   Other_____

HEAD AND NECK (Figure 4-16—see page 114)

Procedure:	• *Radical neck dissection:* A major procedure that involves excision of a tumor in the neck region, including the lymph node network. It is the most frequently used procedure. • *Commando procedure:* Includes the resection of part of the mandible.
Perioperative care:	Dissection and resection in the neck region may involve removal of portions of the oral cavity floor, the palate, larynx, and thyroid, depending on the degree of involvement. A temporary or permanent tracheostomy may be constructed. Drain catheters are placed and connected to suction to eliminate collection of fluid under the flaps and to prevent respiratory complications.

Postoperative nursing care

1. The patient will spend the initial postoperative period in the ICU for close observation.
2. You must be competent in caring for a patient with a tracheostomy. The patient requires frequent suctioning, oxygen, and high humidity therapy and must be closely observed for signs and symptoms of respiratory distress. An extra tracheostomy set should always be taped to the head of the bed, and there should be an extra tracheostomy tray in the patient's room.
3. Alternative forms of communicating with the patient should be provided, such as pad of paper and a pencil, at the patient's bedside. If the tracheostomy is permanent, a speech therapist will assist you and the patient in learning a new method of speaking.

FIGURE 4-15 NURSING THE THYROIDECTOMY PATIENT

Pre-op teaching

1. Teach patient how to support neck after surgery when getting up or returning to bed (hands clasped behind occipital area to prevent strain on suture line).
2. Deep breathing only (no coughing), unless otherwise instructed, for the first 24-hours post-op.
3. Will have some hoarseness for about 24 hours (sometimes longer); also some difficulty swallowing for a few days.
4. May have high humidity face mask (HHFM).
5. Inform patient of symptoms of hypocalcemia; instruct patient to notify nurse immediately if he has any symptoms.
6. Serum calcium levels may be drawn one or two times per day (more important for total thyroidectomy).

Potential problems	Nursing intervention or management	Outcome
● Shock secondary to: a. anesthesia b. blood loss	1. VS per recovery room routine then qh for four hours, q4h for first day, then bid if stable. 2. Check dressing or incision (check for drainage behind neck) with each VS check. If dressing needs reinforcing, notify surgeon, as drainage should be minimal. 3. Check skin color, turgor, temp, and integrity. Check LOC and mental acuity.	1. Documentation of VS. 2. Documentation of dressing condition q shift until removed, then documentation of condition of incision line bid until discharge. Incision line intact, clean, and dry at time of discharge.
● Respiratory distress secondary to: a. edema of glottis b. swelling of tissue surrounding trachea c. local hemorrhage causing compression of trachea d. pneumothorax	1. Observe respiration as per above. 2. Observe for: a. rapid, shallow, noisy respirations b. swelling in incisional area c. increased difficulty with swallowing d. restlessness, confusion e. pallor, cyanosis f. ↓ BP, ↑ P. *Precautions:* 1. Trach tray at bedside first 24 hours per doctor's order. 2. Head of bed elevated 30° or higher. 3. HHFM for 24 hours, per doctor's order.	1. Documentation if respiratory distress develops that physician was notified immediately. 2. Documentation that trach tray is at bedside. No episodes of respiratory distress post-op.

- Pneumonia secondary to:
  a. anesthesia
  b. immobility
  c. hypoventilation

1. Check temperature q4h for first 24 hours, then q6h for next 24 hours, then bid (more often if temp > 99.6°).
2. Turn and deep breathe q2h for 24 hours (q4h at night). Encourage coughing after first 24 hours (blow glove or incentive spirometer, per doctor's order).
3. Activity:
   a. Up to bathroom or up at bedside the evening of surgery.
   b. Ambulate at least qid (from first POD until discharge).
4. HHFM, per doctor's order, first 24 hours, to loosen secretions.

1. Documentation that physician was notified of temp > 101°.
2. Documentation of turning and deep breathing q2h for first 24 hours.
3. Documentation that patient is ambulatory at least qid 24 hours prior to discharge.
4. Lungs clear at time of discharge.
5. Temp < 99.6° at time of discharge.

- Hypocalcemia or tetany secondary to:
  a. incidental removal of parathyroids
  b. trauma to parathyroids

1. Check for symptoms of hypocalcemia.
   a. General symptoms:
      1) irritability
      2) circumoral tingling
      3) muscle twitching
      4) cramping in legs or abdomen
      5) numbness or tingling in extremities
      6) sometimes nausea and vomiting.
      7) carpopedal spasm (contraction of thumb and fingers and inability to open hand)
   b. Chvostek's sign: tapping anterior to the external ear and immediately below the temporal bone over the facial nerve causes a twitch of the lip or facial muscles.
   c. Trousseau's sign: inflating the BP cuff slightly above the systolic BP for three minutes initiates carpopedal spasm.

Documentation that numbness or tingling in extremities is absent q4h for the first 24 hours post-op then bid and prn.

No episode of tetany convulsions.

If any of general symptoms present, documentation that physician is notified immediately, and check Chvostek's and Trousseau's signs and document results.

Continued on next page.

FIGURE 4-15 continued

Potential problems	Nursing intervention or management	Outcome
	2. Check serum calcium level bid or as ordered and mark requisition to be done ASAP. Notify physician if patient has low serum calcium or is symptomatic. *Precautions:* 1. Ampule of IV calcium at bedside. 2. Physician may order IV—TKO for 24 to 48 hours in case patient needs IV administration of calcium.	Patient maintains normal serum calcium (9.0–10.6 mg/dl). Documentation of low serum calcium, notification of physician, and any intervention initiated.
• Injury to recurrent laryngeal nerve	Ask patient to speak qid. Note any changes in voice. Expect some hoarseness post-op. Assess for progression of symptoms; it may indicate possible damage.	Documentation of quality of voice q8h for first 24 hours. Patient discharged with normal speaking voice.
• Wound infection	1. Check incision for redness, swelling, drainage, separation. 2. Check temp as above. 3. Incisions should be kept dry. Sutures are usually removed second POD and steristrips applied. May shower and pat incision dry after first 24 hours (varies with surgeon).	Documentation that temp < 99.6° for 24 hours prior to discharge. Documentation of appearance of suture line.

- Thyroid storm secondary to manipulation of gland during surgery (only with subtotal thyroidectomy)

This is a medical emergency (usually within 24 hours post-op), though rare.

1. Symptoms
   a. severe tachycardia
   b. fever
   c. extreme irritability
   d. delirium
   e. diarrhea
2. All treatment per doctor's orders. May give:
   1. Na⁺ iodine IV (inhibits release of hormone from thyroid)
   2. propanolol
   3. other symptomatic treatment

Discharge instructions:
1. If total thyroidectomy, will need to take thyroid medication for rest of life.
2. May shower.
3. If hypocalcemia persists, will go home on oral supplement and/or vitamin D. Instruct patient again about symptoms of hypocalcemia.
4. Activity as per physician's direction.

Documentation that if symptoms of thyroid storm occurred physician was notified immediately.

Documentation that patient has received discharge instruction and is able to verbalize them.

FIGURE 4-16 NURSING THE PATIENT WITH RADICAL NECK DISSECTION

Pre-op teaching

1. If a patient is to have a total laryngectomy:
   a. Discuss alternative means of communication to be utilized during the post-op period (pen and paper, small chalkboard, magic slate).
   b. Arrange a pre-op visit by a speech therapist or laryngectomy visitor.
2. Discuss surgical drains, short-term need for tube feedings.
3. Instruct patient on deep breathing exercises with emphasis on possible presence of tracheostomy tube and suction procedure; how to handle cough and secretions.

Potential problems	Nursing intervention or management	Outcome
• Obstruction of airway secondary to: a. local edema b. local hemorrhage c. tracheostomy tube displacement	1. Observe for restlessness, dyspnea, tachycardia, confusion. 2. Check rate and quality of respirations. 3. Check skin color for cyanosis, pallor. 4. Observe any increase of swelling in neck region/incisional area. 5. Observe for a change in VS. 6. Monitor blood gas results. 7. Have head of bed raised 30° or higher. 8. Keep trach tray at bedside. If patient has a trach tube in place, also have a replacement—same type, size, with all pieces—at bedside.	1. Documentation of any respiratory distress. 2. Documentation that physician was notified immediately. 3. Patient has no respiratory distress.
• Hemorrhage secondary to: a. carotid artery blowout b. anastomotic leak	1. Take VS frequently. 2. Observe suture line for disruption, discoloration of area, drainage. 3. Check dressing and drain tubes frequently for color, amount. 4. If hemorrhage occurs, direct pressure is applied until patient goes to OR.	1. Documentation of excessive drainage, change in VS. 2. Documentation that physician was notified immediately. 3. No hemorrhage.

Potential problems	Nursing intervention or management	Outcome
• Delayed healing and/or wound infection. Patient who has undergone radiation treatments prior to surgery will be at increased risk.	1. Check temperature. 2. Observe integrity of suture line. 3. Check dressings, suture line for purulent, foul-smelling drainage.	1. Documentation of elevated temperature, dressing changes, presence and description of drainage. 2. Complete healing of suture line.
• Nutrition	1. During initial post-op period, a feeding tube is inserted. 2. Tube feedings are administered according to physician's order. Initially, feedings are started in small amounts and then increased according to patient's tolerance. 3. Head of bed should be elevated to promote digestion and prevent aspiration. 4. Oral feedings will be started once adequate healing occurs. Patient starts with small amounts of clear liquids and then progresses. Patient may be discharged from the hospital on tube feeding, in which case he and family members must be instructed on the mechanics of tube feeding and what precautions to take. 5. Check for development of diarrhea. If it occurs, change type of feeding, administer corrective medication, or take other appropriate measures.	1. Documentation of tube feeding and patient's tolerance. 2. Documentation that patient understands teaching. 3. No complication of tube feeding administration. 4. Stabilization of weight, good skin. Patient adequately nourished. Documentation of teaching process. Patient or responsible person can demonstrate correct tube feeding procedure. Patient or responsible person can describe possible complications and corrective action.

Continued on next page.

FIGURE 4-16 continued

Potential problems	Nursing intervention or management	Outcome

• Care of stoma with permanent laryngectomy	1. Observe for development of stenosis of the stoma.
	2. Trach tube may be left in place if:
	  a. Secretions are excessive.
	  b. Stoma tends to close.
	3. Instruct the patient on:
	  a. Care of trach tube.
	  b. How to cough and expectorate secretions.
	  c. How to clean stoma area.
	  d. Importance of good skin care.
	  e. Danger of inserting any object into the stoma.
	  f. Importance of humidity, to avoid extremes in temperature.
		1. Documentation that patient understands teaching.
		2. Patient is able to care for stoma, tubes independently. Patient or responsible person can describe proper stoma care and precautions and perform demonstration of them.

• Communication	1. During initial post-op period, help with use of alternative means of communication—pen/paper, small chalkboard, magic slate.
	2. Patient to learn esophageal speech pattern, if possible:
	  a. Instruction and follow-up with speech therapist.
	  b. Visit from person with a laryngectomy.
	  c. Need for care givers and family to be understanding and supportive.
		1. Documentation of teaching process.
		2. Patient usually discharged prior to completion of speech training.
		3. Documentation of referral or arrangements for follow-up care.

4. Nutrition is an important postoperative consideration. The patient has a feeding tube inserted as an alternative to eating. The primary nurse may need to teach the patient and family how to perform tube feedings if the patient is to be discharged before oral consumption of food is resumed.
5. The patient who has undergone a radical neck dissection has experienced major alterations, whether temporary or permanent, in two vital functions: breathing and eating. It is important that you provide emotional support and reassurance by finding ways for the patient's expression of feelings about these alterations and that you ensure adequate respiratory function and nutrition.

KIDNEY, BLADDER (Figure 4-17—see page 118)

Procedure:
- *Nephrectomy:* Removal of the kidney.
- *Cystectomy:* Removal of the bladder.
- *Ureteroileostomy* (ileal conduit): Removal of the bladder with creation of urinary diversion.

Perioperative: Two major types of urinary diversions may be constructed:

Cutaneous ureterostomy. The ureters are brought to the skin surface. Two stomas may be constructed, or the ureter may be connected into a loop and one stoma created. Temporary stent catheters may be inserted into one or both ureters to assure patency during the immediate postoperative period.

Ileal conduit. A 6-8 cm segment of the ileum is resected above the ileocecal valve, and the ureters are anatomosed into this segment. The distal portion is brought to the surface, and a stoma is constructed. The stoma may protrude onto the abdomen or it may be flush with the skin.

Postoperative nursing care

1. Appliances used differ in some aspects from those used for the colostomy patient. The importance of fit and teaching the patient self-care are the same.
2. Skin protection and the importance of good seal with the appliance are imperative for the patient who has had a urinary diversion, because urine is a potent skin irritant. Frequent cleansing of the area around the stoma is essential.
3. Urine collects in the pouch, which postoperatively is connected to a urinary drainage system similar to a Foley catheter. Prior to

FIGURE 4-17 NURSING THE NEPHRECTOMY PATIENT

Potential problems	Nursing intervention or management	Outcome
• Renal shutdown of opposite kidney	Monitor urine output; it should be 30 cc or more per hour.	Urine output > 30 cc/hour.
• Hemorrhage	1. Monitor VS. 2. Note dressings for increased drainage and notify service immediately of unusually large amounts.	Absence of hemorrhage.
• Infection	1. Monitor temperature. 2. Antibiotic therapy usually ordered for initial post-op period. Drug frequency and length of administration depend on physician's preference. 3. Check dressing, suture line for purulent, foul-smelling drainage, amount. 4. Surgical/incisional drains normally placed during time of surgery.	Normal temperature and no other signs of infection.
• Pneumonia	1. Teach coughing and deep breathing and turn. 2. Start ambulation early. 3. Make use of artificial ventilation. 4. Note signs of increased respiratory distress. Tumor may be located near diaphragm or diaphragm may be affected by resection.	No respiratory complications.

discharge, the drainage system is changed and the patient is fitted with a pouch in which urine collects. The pouch must be periodically emptied.

4. Adequate oral fluid intake is essential to prevent urinary tract infection.

5. To control odor, good hygiene and proper cleansing and changing of pouches are essential. The patient should be informed about causes of odor such as certain drugs, foods, or infection.

REPRODUCTIVE SYSTEM (Figures 4-18—see page 120 and 4-19—see page 122)

Procedure:

- *Transurethral resection of the prostate:* An endoscope is passed through the penis to visualize the prostate and then resect the tissue. After removal is complete, a catheter is inserted and is usually connected to an irrigation setup (Figure 4-20). Sample nursing procedures for bladder irrigation are provided in Figures 4-21 and 4-22.

- *Suprapubic prostatectomy:* The removal of the prostate tissue through a longitudinal incision. The bladder is filled, which results in compression of the prostate. The prostate and the prostatic urethra are resected. A suprapubic catheter is then inserted with or without connection to an irrigation setup.

- *Orchiectomy:* The removal of the testis, usually performed through the inguinal approach (as with the repair of a hernia). The spermatic vessels are examined and a clip is placed on the cord. Resection occurs with a metal clip remaining in place to serve as marker for additional surgery or radiation.

- *Hysterectomy:* A **vaginal approach** is preferred in some females if a safe, thorough resection can occur. In the presence of a large uterus or large tumor mass, the abdominal approach is utilized. The **abdominal approach** is carried out through an abdominal incision. In younger patients, every attempt is made to leave at least one ovary and tube intact if

Continued on page 125.

FIGURE 4-18 NURSING THE PATIENT WITH
TRANSURETHRAL RESECTION OF THE PROSTATE

Pre-op teaching

1. Explain to patient that postoperatively he will have a catheter connected to an irrigation setup.
2. Explain post-op hematuria.
3. Review pain medication and warn that irrigation will create discomfort.

Potential problems	Nursing intervention or management	Outcome
• Hemorrhage secondary to blood loss	1. Check VS q15 min for two hours, then qh for four hours, then q2h for the next 24 hours. 2. Observe drainage via Foley catheter. 3. Irrigate according to established procedures (see Figure 4-23). 4. Observe for difficulty in irrigation, increased pain. 5. Monitor post-op hgb, hct.	1. Documentation of drainage, irrigation, presence of clots. 2. No evidence of hemorrhage.
• Electrolyte imbalance	1. Keep accurate record of intake and output. Subtract irrigation fluid from urine output to monitor "true urine output." 2. Initial fluids IV with gradual resumption of PO intake. 3. Check for patency of catheter (indicated by decreased urine output). Patient may express urgency to void or increased discomfort. a. Check output. b. Irrigate.	1. Documentation of output with notes on color, consistency, amount, presence of clots. 2. Return to normal intake/output and electrolyte balance.

Potential problems	Nursing intervention or management	Outcome
● Bladder spasms	1. Observe for intermittent episodes of severe discomfort. 2. Use of antispasmodic medication prn (propantheline, belladonna, opium suppositories).	No occurrence of bladder spasms.
● Return of normal bladder function	1. Catheter is removed, usually 3–5 days post-op. 2. Note and record first void after catheter removal for color, amount, and presence of clots. 3. If patient unable to void six hours after catheter removal, notify service. It may be necessary to reinsert the catheter.	1. Documentation of catheter removal, time of first voiding. 2. Documentation of return of normal color of urine without the presence of clots. 3. Normal bladder function without complications.

Discharge instructions should include:

a. Restrictions on bending, lifting, driving.
b. Preventive measures against constipation.
c. Physician's instructions regarding resumption of sexual activity (varies according to procedure, extent of surgery, and patient).

FIGURE 4-19 NURSING THE HYSTERECTOMY PATIENT

Potential problems	Nursing intervention or management	Outcome
• Shock secondary to blood loss, anesthesia, fluid loss	1. Check VS qh for six hours, then q4h for 24 hours, then bid. 2. Check perineal pad qh for six hours, then bid. Notify service if more than two pads are needed in eight hours, or if patient has vaginal pack and saturates more than one pad in eight hours.	1. Stabilization of vital signs. 2. Documentation of amount of drainage and, if excessive, of notification of physician.
• Pain secondary to surgery	1. Pain medication offered q3-4h prn or more often if necessary and/or ordered. 2. Patients who have A & P repair complain of increased pain secondary to pressure on bladder from vaginal pack. Be sure to check that Foley is patent.	Patient verbalizes reasonable control of pain.
• Dehydration	1. NPO if ordered; ice chips if allowed. 2. Record intake and output until IV and Foley catheter discontinued and intake/output satisfactory. 3. Encourage fluids when patient is back on diet.	1. Balanced state of hydration. 2. Documentation of input and output.

Potential problems	Nursing intervention or management	Outcome
• Pneumonia secondary to anesthesia, immobility; venous stasis or thrombus formation secondary to decreased activity	1. Turning, coughing and deep breathing q2h for first 24 hours. 2. First POD, up in chair qid or to bathroom with assistance. 3. Second POD, ambulating in room or hall if tolerated. Patient with vaginal hysterectomy may shower, if stable, and IV out; patient with abdominal hysterectomy on third POD if stable. 4. No dangling legs from side of bed; no pillow under knees in bed. Antiembolism stockings if ordered.	1. Clear lungs; no atelectasis or pneumonia. 2. Documentation of breath sounds. 3. Patient ambulating with minimal assistance by third POD. 4. Documentation of application and wearing of stockings.
• Trauma to bladder secondary to surgical procedure; urinary tract infection	1. Check that Foley catheter is taped to leg at all times with slack in tube. 2. Check quality and quantity of urine q1-2h for eight hours, then q8h. Notify service if gross hematuria present. 3. Catheter care bid and prn: a. Maintain closed system. b. Wash area around Foley and meatus with soap and water during A.M. care. c. Using clean gloves and 4 x 4's, cleanse urinary meatus, catheter, and perineum with Betadine solution bid.	No urinary tract infection. Documentation of catheter care.

Continued on next page.

FIGURE 4-19 continued

Potential problems	Nursing intervention or management	Outcome

	4. Fluid intake:
	  a. When tolerating fluids, offer cranberry juice qid to keep urine acidic and decrease infection.
	  b. Encourage fluids to 3000 cc day.
	5. When Foley discontinued, check with doctor about further catheter orders.
		Adequate hydration. Patient has adequate urinary output.

• Vaginal vault or incisional infection secondary to surgical procedure	1. Temp q4h for first 24 hours, then qid for three days, then bid.	No post-op vault or incisional infection.
• Abdominal distension and discomfort secondary to gas or paralytic ileus	1. For gas pains, ambulate and/or put hot water bottle to abdomen or rectal tube if ordered (not used for A & P repairs). 2. Suppository or enema as ordered. 3. Check abdomen for distension and passing of flatus q shift. Record all stools.	Passing flatus by third to fourth POD.
• Emotional problems secondary to surgery, change in body image, hormonal changes	1. Reassure patient. 2. Allow patient to verbalize. 3. Give pre-op explanation about post-op course and continue to teach patient about what to expect psychologically and physically post-op and after discharge.	Patient feels free to verbalize feelings, is able to verbalize pre-op and post-op teaching.

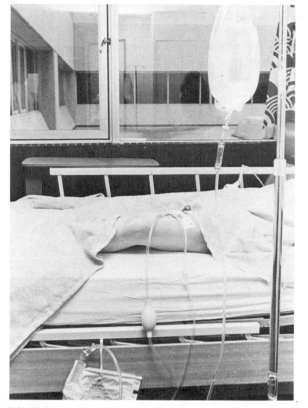

FIGURE 4-20. URINARY CATHETER CONNECTED TO AN
IRRIGATION SETUP.

there is no sign of further spread of the
malignancy. However, in most patients a
bilateral salpingo-oophorectomy is carried out
to prevent metastases. The uterus is
identified and the bladder is separated from
the uterus and cervix. Extreme caution must
be taken not to injure the bladder, ureters, or
intestines. After removal is completed, the
next step is pelvic reconstruction to provide
temporary support to the vagina until healing
is accomplished.

- *Total abdominal hysterectomy:* Removal of
  the uterus, ovaries, and fallopian tubes.
- *Pelvic exenteration:* Removal of the uterus,
  ovaries, fallopian tubes, bladder, and bowel.

FIGURE 4-21 CLOSED SYSTEM BLADDER IRRIGATION

Purpose:	1. To prevent or relieve plugging of catheter.
	2. To cleanse bladder.
Equipment:	1. 1000 cc bag irrigating solution.
	2. Irrigating tubing.
	3. Foley adapter.
	4. Hemostat.
	5. IV pole.
Actions:	1. Assemble equipment with careful regard to sterile technique.

        a. Clamp tubing and attach to bag. Place bag on IV pole and remove air from tubing.

        b. Clamp Foley. Attach Foley adapter to end of Foley and to end of drainage tubing.

        c. Attach irrigating tubing to Foley adapter.

        d. Unclamp Foley.

    2. Irrigation.

        a. Clamp drainage tubing with hemostat.

        b. Unclamp irrigating tubing and allow 50 cc of solution to slowly flow into bladder if patient can tolerate this amount. Then clamp irrigating tubing.

        c. Unclamp drainage tubing and note returns.

    3. Charting.

        a. Subtract amount of irrigating solution used from the total output from Foley bag.

        b. Record character of drainage in the progress notes.

Postoperative nursing care

1. A major postoperative consideration is assisting the patient to deal with alteration of body image due to the removal of the reproductive organs. These operations, obviously, have a profound impact on sexual function, and for those of childbearing age they mean loss of the ability to reproduce. Patients may experience feelings of loss of masculinity or femininity. For example, if surgery involves radical procedures, a penile prosthesis may assist in the male's psychological readjustment, just as breast reconstruction helps the woman. Following salpingo-oophorectomy, hormonal replacement is necessary.

2. In the male, there may be numerous different types of drains inserted and special irrigation procedures.

3. The female patient may undergo radiation treatment with implantation of radium as part of therapy.

FIGURE 4-22 BLADDER IRRIGATION AFTER
TRANSURETHRAL RESECTION OF THE PROSTATE

Purpose:	1. Prevent accumulation of blood clots in bladder. 2. Keep the bladder empty (a distended bladder promotes postoperative bleeding).
Equipment:	1. Foley 2. 3000 cc. bag irrigating solution. 3. Irrigating tubing with Foley adapter. 4. IV pole. 5. Sterile basin. 6. 50 cc catheter-irrigating syringe. 7. 1000 cc bottle of irrigating solution.
Action:	1. The catheter may have traction applied and be taped to the thigh to compress the bladder neck and tamponade prostatic bleeding. Therefore, blood may exude around catheter at meatus. Cleanse this area frequently (use one-half strength peroxide) and apply Betadine Ointment. 2. The irrigation system allows gravity drainage of normal saline in and out of bladder intermittently. There may be a rubber bulb on the outlet drainage tubing to syringe out clots. Occlude below bulb, run in solution, squeeze bulb and release several times. This also allows you to confirm that catheter is not blocked by clot. And the system remains sterile and closed because you have not disconnected anything. 3. It should be apparent if catheter is blocked by clot, because irrigation into bladder fails or it is not followed by rapid drainage out of bladder. 4. If catheter is blocked and cannot be unplugged, you can, using the bulb in the drainage tube, disconnect the catheter aseptically and irrigate the catheter with catheter-irrigating syringe (2 oz piston). Inject fluid into the bladder and aspirate. If this fails to establish completely free drainage which is not bloodier than a pink color, call service stat. A plugged catheter in a transurethral resection patient is an emergency situation. 5. The catheter should be irrigated to test for obstruction every 15 minutes after a transurethral resection if the drainage is bright red or thick or if there are clots. The above-described irrigations are employed. If the bleeding is red but not thick and there are no clots, do the irrigations every 30 minutes. If the drainage is pink, irrigate every one or two hours. If it is clear or faintly colored red—if you're suspicious of obstruction—irrigate prn. 6. The patient will sense an urge to void even if the catheter is patent. This is due to bladder spasm and it is painful. Give pain medication, but first be certain catheter is not plugged. 7. Subtract the used amount of irrigating fluid from the patient's output.

PITUITARY GLAND (Figures 4-23 and 4-24— see pages 129 and 130)

Procedure:

- *Transsphenoidal hypophysectomy:* The surgical removal of the pituitary gland utilizing an approach through the upper lip, the nasal passage, and the sphenoid sinus.

Perioperative note:

- This procedure is executed with the assistance of special operative microscopes and fluoroscopy to allow for good visualization. This technique is usually utilized when the tumors are small and confined to the sella turcica. A piece of muscle tissue is usually removed from the thigh and grafted to cover the space left by removal of the pituitary gland.

Postoperative considerations:

1. Replacement hormone therapy is administered. Corticosteroids are given, and mineralocorticoids may also be initiated for short- or long-term supplement. Also, other hormones must be replaced, including thyroid, androgens for men, and estrogens in premenopausal women.
2. It is important to maintain proper fluid and electrolyte balance. Patients may experience transient diabetes insipidus, and it is important that you observe urine output with initial frequent checks of the specific gravity. In these cases, antidiuretic hormone may be supplemented; some patients may require long-term therapy.
3. The patient has nasal packing in place with a small "moustache" dressing on the upper lip. Check these dressings frequently for drainage.
4. It is important that you be aware of the serious nature an infection poses in this postoperative patient. Immediately report any sign of unusual foul-smelling drainage or an increased temperature.

FIGURE 4-23 CONSIDERATIONS FOR HYPOPHYSECTOMY PATIENTS

Learning needs	Patient education	Evaluation
• Anxiety about disease process	Assess patient's knowledge of disease and expectations about surgery.	Reduction of anxiety by meeting identified patient needs.
• Blocks to learning: a. pain b. unrealistic expectations of surgery	1. Keep as comfortable as possible prior to surgery with appropriate analgesic and comfort measures.	Patient as comfortable as possible
	2. Gear teaching to patient's emotional and physical tolerance.	Patient taught to limits of emotional and physical tolerance.
	3. Discuss patient's expectations of surgery. Evaluate understanding of physician's teaching and reinforce the teaching.	Patient understands possibility of pain reductions but does not view procedure as a cure for disease process.
• Nutritional status	1. Keep accurate intake and output records and/or daily weights. 2. Encourage food and fluid intake. 3. Observe for anemia.	Adequate nutritional status to tolerate surgery.

• Skin breakdown	1. Ensure frequent changes of position.
	2. Provide alternating pressure mattress or water mattress.
	3. Ensure adequate hydration. Employ skin care measures:
	  a. lanolin preparations for bath
	  b. back care
	  c. check for pressure areas
		Absence of skin breakdown or improvement of pre-existing breakdown.

• Family difficulty in dealing with disease process and/or surgical procedure	1. Assess family's level of acceptance of patient's illness and outcome of surgery. 2. Involve patient's family in the educational process. 3. Involve family in patient's care if appropriate.	Family has realistic comprehension of illness. Family has been included in educational process.

FIGURE 4-24 TEACHING THE PRE-OP HYPOPHYSECTOMY PATIENT

Learning needs	Patient education	Evaluation
• Simple explanation of location and the function of pituitary	Show patient picture of pituitary and surrounding structures. For information on function, refer to any standard text.	Patient can give verbal feedback regarding location and function of pituitary. ☐ Yes ☐ No
• Explanation of pathophysiology of patients with pituitary disorders.	Identify abnormal hormonal secretion and its effects. Refer to any standard text for information on effects of abnormal hormone secretion.	Patient will be able to give verbal feedback regarding his own specific problem. ☐ Yes ☐ No
• Explanation of diagnostic tests and procedures	Refer to any standard text.	Patient can give verbal feedback on purpose and procedure of tests. Tests have been successfully carried out. ☐ Yes ☐ No
• Simple explanation of operative procedure	Teach patient about: 1. Location of incision under lip. 2. Purpose of incision on thigh and muscle packing. 3. Nasal pack and mustache dressing.	Patient can enumerate number and location of incisions and dressings. ☐ Yes ☐ No
• Pre-op preparation	1. Arrange for patient to meet another hypophysectomized patient. 2. Use antibiotic nose drops and antibiotics PO. 3. Administer loading doses of steroids to cover through stress of surgery. 4. Instruct patient to mouth breathe (pinch nostrils) and drink with straw.	 Patient can demonstrate correct mouth breathing. ☐ Yes ☐ No

Learning needs	Patient education	Evaluation
• Post-op expectations	In addition to routine post-op procedures, information to be discussed specific to this surgery includes: 1. Routine early recovery in ICU. 2. Flat position or raised no more than 30° for at least 48 hours; no bending over. 3. Frequent checking of neurological signs. 4. Frequent testing of urine specific gravity. 5. Accurate recording of intake and output. 6. Availability of antiemetics if nauseated. 7. No sneezing and coughing. If sneeze is unavoidable, keep mouth open.	Patient can describe routine post-op procedures. ☐ Yes ☐ No Patient can explain reasons for no sneezing or coughing. ☐ Yes ☐ No
	8. Possibility of permanent or temporary replacement of hormones.	Patient understands possibility of permanent or temporary hormone replacement post-op. ☐ Yes ☐ No
	9. Temporary changes in facial appearance; various degrees of facial edema and bruising post-up.	Patient understands that temporary facial changes will result. ☐ Yes ☐ No

BIBLIOGRAPHY

Bates B. A GUIDE TO PHYSICAL EXAMINATION, 3rd ed. Philadelphia: Lippincott, 1983.

Beyers M and Dudas S. THE CLINICAL PRACTICE OF MEDICAL-SURGICAL NURSING, 2nd ed. Boston: Little, Brown, 1984.

Broodwell D and Jackson B (eds). PRINCIPLES OF OSTOMY CARE. St Louis: Mosby, 1982.

CLINICAL ONCOLOGY FOR MEDICAL STUDENTS AND PHYSICIANS: A MULTIDISCIPLINARY APPROACH, 6th ed. Rochester, NY: University of Rochester School of Medicine/Dentistry, 1983.

Del Regato JA and Spjut HJ. ACKERMAN AND DEL REGATO'S CANCER: DIAGNOSIS, TREATMENT, AND PROGNOSIS, 5th ed. St Louis: Mosby, 1977.

Luckmann J and Sorensen KC. MEDICAL-SURGICAL NURSING: A PSYCHOPHYSIOLOGIC APPROACH, 2nd ed. Philadelphia: Saunders, 1980.

Moss T, Brond WN, and Batifore H. RADIATION ONCOLOGY: RATIONALE, TECHNIQUE, RESULTS, 5th ed. St Louis: Mosby, 1979.

Schwartz SI, Shirer GT, Spencer FC, et al. PRINCIPLES OF SURGERY, 3rd ed. New York: McGraw-Hill, 1979.

STANDARD CARE PLANS. Evanston, Ill: Evanston Hospital Corporation, 1983.

Woods ME and Kowalski JD (eds). A symposium on oncologic nursing practice. NURS CLIN NORTH AM 17:535, 1982.

5
CHEMOTHERAPY

SUSAN B. ANDERSON, RN, BSN

There are many anticancer drugs both in use and under investigation. It would be difficult to describe all of them here. This chapter includes information about drugs used most frequently for cancer treatment, their more commonly encountered side effects, the nurse's role in chemotherapy, how it affects the individual patient, and how to use the nursing process to provide care that is responsive to all of the patient's needs.

Chemotherapy is the use of drugs to destroy cancer cells with minimal toxicity to healthy cells. The goal of this systemic treatment may be to eliminate the disease or to palliate metastatic disease to prolong survival and improve the quality of an individual patient's life. To date, there is no one drug that can effectively destroy cancer cells without affecting normal cellular function. For that reason, nurses and physicians plan and implement a program of chemotherapy for each cancer patient individually.

Knowing about the cell cycle is essential to understanding tumor growth and the principles of chemotherapy. The cell cycle consists of two periods, interphase and mitosis. Cellular growth takes place during interphase. The cycle can also be divided into five specific phases as follows:

G_1—enzymes necessary for DNA production are generated; cell enlarges. Duration is variable.

S—DNA is synthesized. Duration is 10–12 hours.

G_2—specialized protein and RNA are synthesized. Duration is two to 10 hours.

M—mitosis occurs. Duration is one-half to one hour.

G_0—resting phase; cell is not committed to division at this time. Duration is variable.

Mitosis is the short time during which the cell actually divides into two cells, the parent cell and daughter cell. It consists of four stages:

Prophase—chromosomes begin to "clump."

Metaphase—chromosomes begin to line up in the center of the cell.

Anaphase—chromosomes segregate to the centrioles.

Telephase—cellular division.

Cancer cells often spend a longer time in the actual process of cell division; therefore, malignant tissue has a greater percentage of cells undergoing division at a given time.

The number of tumor cells in the division stage depends on the type of malignancy. Most tumors have a high growth fraction when the tumor is young and small and a low growth fraction later when it is large. The high rate of cellular proliferation makes malignant tissues more susceptible to chemotherapy. Unfortunately, healthy cells with a high growth index can be affected by these drugs, which produce toxic side effects.

The administration of chemotherapeutic drugs

How chemotherapy is administered depends upon the drug being used and the disease being treated. The following is a list of the various routes of administration:

- intravenous,
- intra-arterial,
- intramuscular,
- intrathecal (into the CSF by lumbar puncture or through an Omaya reservoir*),

---

*Omaya reservoir is a spongelike plate surgically implanted in the skull that provides direct access to a specific brain site. Component parts are a self-sealing Silastic dome and a catheter that is inserted into the ventricle on the patient's nondominant side. This allows for direct access to the CNS without repeated lumbar punctures.

- intracavity (directly into a cavity, such as bladder),
- subcutaneous,
- oral, and
- topical.

The equipment used varies with each drug and method of administration. Procedures for administration vary in different care settings. For example, drugs such as doxorubicin (Adriamycin) or mitomycin-C, which, when given intravenously, have a potential for extravasation and consequent tissue necrosis, may be given through a buret chamber, pushed through a rapid-flowing IV line, or simply given "push" followed by a flush with saline or sterile water. The use of a buret chamber allows for the drug to be further diluted so that if an infiltration should occur, the toxicity to the local tissue is minimized. On the other hand, the "push" method may allow for a quicker assessment of a possible infiltration while allowing access to the site with a free-flowing IV line. It is thought by some that the intravenous pressure exerted by a "push" may enhance an infiltration.

Venous access is often a problem with patients receiving chemotherapy. Frequency of treatment may be five times a week, but even if it is not that often, venipuncture for blood tests and drug administration becomes difficult, uncomfortable, and unsafe. Long-term indwelling catheters are helpful for patients with poor venous access. Patients with indwelling catheters must learn how to manage the catheter. Management includes daily heparin injections and weekly dressing changes. It is not unknown for the same indwelling catheter to remain in place for 21 months without complications.

The preparation of the drugs may be done by pharmacists or nurses, depending upon the institution. Each drug should be reconstituted according to directions and under a laminar flow system. Whoever prepares the drugs should wear gloves and avoid direct contact with the chemicals. To date, very little is known about the potential short- and long-term hazards of drug exposure. For disposal, it's recommended that the drugs and containers be burned to prevent contamination of the surrounding environment.

It is important that each institution develop specific procedures and guidelines for administering chemotherapy, to assure correct procedures in preparation and administration of chemotherapeutic agents, and to protect the patient and the staff.

Classes of chemotherapy agents

An overview of chemotherapeutic agents is shown in Table 5-1. The following are descriptions of each class of agent.

Alkylating agents. The alkylating agents are highly reactive compounds with the ability to substitute alkyl groups for hydrogen atoms. The major effect appears to be cross-linking of DNA strands by covalent bonding of a pair of guanines. As a result, transcription and replication of DNA cannot be completed. Synthesis of RNA, proteins, and other cellular components continues, causing a cellular imbalance and, eventually, cell death. Certain types of radiation can cause similar effects. Therefore, alkylating agents are considered radiomimetic.

Antimetabolites. The antimetabolites work most effectively during the S phase of the cell cycle. These drugs are structural analogues of metabolites that the cell normally uses during replication. There are three ways in which an antimetabolite interferes with cellular function:

- substituting for a metabolite within the molecule;
- competing with a metabolite for a particular site of an enzyme; and
- competing with a metabolite that regulates enzymes, causing the catalytic rate to be altered.

Antitumor antibiotics. The antibiotics are natural products of various strains of the soil fungus *(Streptomyces)*. Most of these drugs have some anti-infective properties, but they are used for their toxic effect on cancer cells. The antitumor antibiotics bind to DNA and prevent DNA and RNA synthesis. They appear to be effective during all phases of the cell cycle.

Plant alkaloids. The alkaloids are derived from the periwinkle plant. Their exact mechanism of action is not completely understood. These drugs seem to cause a metaphase arrest during mitosis by crystalizing the microtubular spindle proteins.[5] The effects of these drugs are cumulative, and after high concentrations are reached, they may begin to prevent protein synthesis. Because microtubular proteins are a significant part of nervous tissue, side effects such as paresthesia, constipation, loss of deep tendon reflexes, and acute jaw pain frequently occur after several doses of these drugs.

Hormonal therapy. Hormone therapy is used to minimize the progression of a hormonally dependent tumor by decreasing the growth fraction. There are several theories about how hormones work in the treatment of cancer. Some tumors appear to require certain hormones in order to survive. Some have hormone receptors, which improve chances for a positive response. Hormones are used to block the receptor protein, which deprives the cell of a hormone growth stimulant, or to alter the environment by using antagonistic steroids.

Common Side Effects

Tissues with rapidly dividing cells are most susceptible to drug toxicities. Examples are bone marrow, hair follicles, and the gastrointestinal tract, including the oral mucosa. Another area for drug toxicity is local tissue surrounding the site used for intravenous administration. Table 5-1 provides a detailed list of specific drug toxicities and appropriate nursing interventions.

EXTRAVASATION

Patients can be significantly affected by a drug's infiltration of surrounding tissue during intravenous administration. Some drugs are classified as irritants, but others are vesicants and can cause local tissue necrosis if given perivenously. Ulceration often erodes tissue much deeper than is apparent and can damage tendons or neurovascular structures, which may result in functional joint impairment. Extravasation can and does occur, no matter how cautious you are. For example, your patient may move involuntarily, thus allowing the vein wall to be punctured so that the drug is delivered outside the vessel. Since extravasation is not always avoidable, it is important to develop an emergency treatment procedure to prevent or reduce tissue damage. The following are procedure guidelines:

1. Explain to the patient initially that the drug can cause tissue damage if it gets outside the vein. Explain that you will check blood return frequently and watch the site. Instruct the patient to report any discomfort.
2. Select a large vein, preferably in the forearm, and rotate sites. Drugs such as doxorubicin should be infused as far from the head and joint spaces as possible.
3. Begin infusion with a free-flowing solution, such as normal saline or dextrose, to test viability of the site. Check blood return.
4. Recognize the signs of extravasation:

   - patient complains of stinging or burning at injection site;
   - no blood return or questionable blood return (if there is a leak above the venipuncture site, blood return will still be obtainable despite infiltration); and
   - swelling at the injection site. *Continued on page 146.*

TABLE 5-1 GUIDE TO CHEMOTHERAPEUTIC AGENTS

Drug	Route of administration	Major toxicities, side effects	Nursing implications [See key at end of table for interpretation of letters]
Alkylating agents interfere with DNA replication by cross-linking existing DNA strands, causing a cellular imbalance and eventually cell death. Cell-cycle nonspecific.[1]			
Cytoxan (cyclophosphamide)	PO, IV	Bone marrow depression (1–2 weeks after dose)	A, B, C, D
		Alopecia	H
		Nausea/vomiting	F
		Mucositis	G
		Hemorrhagic cystitis	E. Instruct patient to observe for and report bloody urine, urinary burning or frequency. Encourage patient on oral Cytoxan to take it during the day and to empty bladder frequently.
DTIC-Dome (dacarbazine)	IV, intra-arterial	Bone marrow depression (2–4 weeks after dose)	A, B, C, D
		Nausea/vomiting	F
		Flu-like symptoms (fever, malaise)	Instruct patient to observe for symptoms, take temperature daily.
		Alopecia (uncommon)	H
		Pain with infusion	K. Dilute DTIC (200 mg/100 ml D5W); give over one-half hour, slowly.
BiCNU (carmustine)	IV	Nausea/vomiting/diarrhea	E, F
		BiCNU (pain with infusion)	K. Dilute BiCNU (100 mg/100 ml D5W) and give slowly.

Drug	Route	Toxicity	Codes
CeeNU (lomustine)	PO	Bone marrow depression (delayed, cumulative with CCNU)	A, B, C, D
Methyl CCNU	PO	Stomatitis Neurotoxicity	G J
Mustargen (mechlorethamine)	IV, intracavitary	Bone marrow depression (1–2 weeks after dose)	A, B, C, D
		Nausea/vomiting (severe)	F. Inform patient of potential severe side effect.
		Extravasation	I. If IV infiltrates, do prompt subcutaneous or intradermal injection with isotonic sodium thiosulfate solution.
Thiotepa (triethylenethiophosphoramide)	IV, intracavitary	Bone marrow depression (5–30 days after dose)	A, B, C, D
Myleran (busulfan)	PO	Bone marrow depression (1–2 weeks after dose)	A, B, C, D
Leukeran (chlorambucil)	PO	Bone marrow depression (begins 3 weeks after dose and continues for up to 10 days)	A, B, C, D
Alkeran (melphalan)	PO	Bone marrow depression (5–30 days after dose)	A, B, C, D

Continued on next page.

TABLE 5-1 continued

Drug	Route of administration	Major toxicities, side effects	Nursing implications [See key at end of table for interpretation of letters]
Platinol (cisplatin)	IV	Bone marrow depression (may be long lasting)	A, B, C, D
		Nausea/vomiting/ diarrhea (severe, immediate)	E, F. Give IV fluids, antiemetic prior to administration. Inform patient of expected nausea/vomiting.
		Mucositis	G
		Renal toxicity	Do creatinine clearance and serum creatinine tests routinely. Administer Mannitol. Encourage fluids, frequent bladder emptying. Assess appearance of urine. Watch electrolyte balance.
		Ototoxicity	Instruct patient to watch for and report any change in hearing.
		Neurotoxicity	J

Antimetabolites interfere with DNA synthesis by substituting themselves for purines and pyrimidines essential for DNA and RNA reproduction, resulting in cell death. Cell-cycle specific.[2]

Drug	Route of administration	Major toxicities, side effects	Nursing implications
Methotrexate	IV, IM, PO, inthrathecal	Bone marrow depression (can occur in 24 hours)	A, B, C, D
		Stomatitis (delayed) Nausea/vomiting/ diarrhea (may be immediate)	E, F
		Skin reactions	Instruct patient to keep skin clean and dry, report any irritation or breakdown, minimize sun exposure.

Drug	Route	Side effect	Nursing actions
		Impaired renal function	E. D. IV hydration. Instruct patient to weigh daily, report changes in urination. Obtain creatinne clearance routinely. Watch electrolyte balance.
Fluorouracil	IV, PO, topical	Nausea/vomiting/diarrhea	E, F
		Stomatitis	G. Assess oral cavity routinely. Institute preventative oral care (rinse with salt water)
Cytosar-U (cytarabine)	IV, SC, intrathecal	Bone marrow depression (9–14 days after dose)	A, B, C, D
		Nausea/vomiting	F
		Stomatitis	G
Thioguanine	PO	Bone marrow depression (5–7 days after dose)	A, B, C, D
		Nausea/vomiting	F
		Stomatitis	G
Purinethol (mercaptopurine)	PO	Bone marrow depression (1–4 weeks after dose)	A, B, C, D
		Nausea/vomiting/diarrhea	E, F
		Stomatitis	G
		Bone marrow depression (1–4 weeks after dose)	A, B, C, D

Continued on next page.

TABLE 5-1 continued

Drug	Route of administration	Major toxicities, side effects	Nursing implications [See key at end of table for interpretation of letters]
Antitumor Antibiotics interfere with DNA and RNA synthesis by directly binding with DNA, causing cell death. Cell-cycle nonspecific.[3]			
Adriamycin (doxorubicin)	IV	Bone marrow depression (10–15 days after dose)	A, B, C, D
		Stomatitis	G
		Nausea/vomiting	F
		Alopecia (will occur 10–15 days after dose)	H. Hair loss experienced almost always. Usually complete hair loss.
		Extravasation	I
		Red urine (beginning 24–48 hours after treatment)	Inform patient of possible red urine from drug.
		Cardiac toxicity (dose-related)	Maximum dose 550 mg/m^2. Maintain assessment of adequate cardiac output, i.e., SOB, output, LOC, edema, apical pulse.
Mutamycin (mitomycin)	IV	Bone marrow depression (4–8 weeks after dose)	A, B, C, D
		Stomatitis	G
		Nausea/vomiting	F
		Alopecia	H
		Extravasation	I
		Nephrotoxicity	E. Assess kidney function, serum creatinine, electrolyte balance. Inform patient to report change in urination or appearance of urine.

Drug	Route	Side Effect	Code	Nursing Interventions
Blenoxane (bleomycin)	IV, SC, IM, intrapleural	Nausea/vomiting/diarrhea	E, F	
		Alopecia	H	
		Skin changes		Assess for changes, such as hyperpigmentation, hyperkeratosis, pruritis, ulceration, vesiculations.
		Chemically induced fever		E. Monitor temperature frequently. Instruct patient to take acetaminophen for fever/chills, and report fever.
		Pulmonary fibrosis (dose-related)		Assess lung sounds, SOB, dyspnea. Instruct patient to report changes in breathing. Encourage deep breathing.
Actinomycin	IV	Nausea/vomiting	F	
		Stomatitis	G	
		Bone marrow depression (1–7 days after dose)	A, B, C, D	
		Skin breakdown is possible if patient has had radiation treatment.		
Streptozocin	IV, intra-arterial	Nausea/vomiting	F	
		Bone marrow depression	A, B, C, D	
		Extravasation	I	
		Nephrotoxicity		E. Assess kidney function, creatinine levels, electrolytes. Instruct patient to report change in urination or appearance of urine.
		Hypoglycemia		Assess signs of hypoglycemia: light-headedness, diaphoresis.

Continued on next page.

TABLE 5-1 continued

Drug	Route of administration	Major toxicities, side effects	Nursing implications [See key at end of table for interpretation of letters]
Plant alkaloids interfere with the cell cycle by crystallizing proteins at the M phase and preventing mitosis. Cell-cycle specific.[3]			
Oncovin (vincristine)	IV	Neurotoxicity (dose-related)	J. This commonly occurs following doses. Assess for neurotoxicity before each treatment and record. Dose usually decreased.
		Extravasation	I
Velban (vinblastine)	IV	Bone marrow depression (7–14 days after dose)	A, B, C, D
		Extravasation	I
		Very irritating to vein	Use large distal veins, dilute drug well, and follow with adequate flush.
		Neurotoxicity	J. See entry for Oncovin.
Hormones: The exact mechanism is unclear, but theories of hormonal effectiveness include altering cellular environment, preventing protein synthesis, and interfering with the cell cycle by suppressing mitosis. Cell-cycle nonspecific.[4]			
Androgens	IM, PO	Nausea/vomiting Fluid retention	F Inform patient of possible fluid retention, weigh daily, assess for edema, lung sounds. Low Na+, High K+ diet.
		Virilization	Inform patient beforehand and assure that it is usually temporary.

Drug	Route	Side effect	Nursing action
Estrogens	PO	Nausea/vomiting	F
		Fluid retention	See entry for androgens.
		Feminization	Inform patient beforehand and assure that it is usually temporary. Assess women for uterine bleeding.
Progestins	IM, PO	Pain on injection	Give IM, Z-track, rotate sites.
		Fluid retention	See entry for androgens.
Corticosteroids		Gastric irritation	Administer after meals. Assess CBC, look for blood in stool.
		Increased susceptibility to infection	Observe for fever, chills; may be masked infection.
		Induced diabetes mellitus	Assess FBS. Inform patient of symptoms: polyurea, polydipsia, polyphagia.

Key

A. Routine blood counts.

B. Bleeding precautions; for example, no aspirin, electric razors; instruct patient to report bleeding, avoid injury.

C. Assess for anemia: SOB, tachycardia, nailbeds, mucous membranes.

D. Promote infection control. Instruct patient to avoid crowds, use good hygiene, report signs of infection.

E. Promote adequate hydration. Patient should drink 12 to 15 glasses of fluid each day.

F. Institute antiemetic therapy and assess effectiveness.

G. Encourage optimal oral hygiene, provide appropriate interventions when stomatitis is present. Maintain ongoing assessment of oral cavity.

H. Prior to treatment, inform patient of expected hair loss.

I. Explain that hair loss is an individual response and is temporary. Suggest that patient use a wig.

L. Provide a rapid-flowing IV, observe venipuncture site throughout administration, check blood return carefully. If extravasation occurs, stop IV immediately, apply ice, and institute appropriate protocol. Instruct patient to apply ice for 24 hours and report any change.

J. Inform patient that drugs may affect the CNS. Symptoms to report include acute jaw pain, paralytic ileus, numbness and tingling in extremities. Assess bowel habits and deep tendon reflexes.

K. Inform patient of possible pain during administration. It helps to dilute the drug well and give slowly, following with an adequate flush. Warm and cool compresses applied to arm during infusion may help. Tapping the vein lightly often overrides the discomfort.

5. Once an infiltration has been confirmed, an emergency procedure should be instituted:

- remove the needle,
- apply ice,
- contact physician,
- inject 100 mg Solu-Cortef subcutaneously into the area of infiltration,
- apply hydrocortisone cream 1% and a sterile dressing, and
- instruct the patient to apply the hydrocortisone cream bid, to apply ice for 10 minutes periodically during the first 24 hours, and to report changes.

6. A weekly assessment should be made.

Clinical experience at the Kellogg Cancer Care Center has indicated that the above procedure has been effective for doxorubicin and mitomycin extravasations. The literature includes conflicting data regarding emergency procedures for drug infiltration, although specific information is known for some agents; for example, nitrogen mustard is neutralized by a solution of sodium bicarbonate and thiosulfate.

ALOPECIA

The normal human scalp is composed of more than 100,000 hairs. Ten to 15 percent are actively growing. These growing hairs are affected by chemotherapy. Many agents tend to decrease the size of the hair bulb, which constricts the hair shaft or causes atrophy of the bulb and hair loss. Fortunately, hair loss is temporary, and once the treatment is completed, hair growth returns to normal. Alopecia usually occurs two to three weeks following the initial dose. The response depends upon the patient and the combination of drugs being used. For example, doxorubicin will cause alopecia in most patients. However, cyclophosphamide (Cytoxan) may cause thinning of the hair, complete hair loss, or no effect on the hair at all.

Several techniques have been used to prevent or minimize alopecia, all of which are controversial. These include the application of ice to the scalp, the use of a scalp tourniquet, and the use of a special scalp sphygmomanometer. The purpose of these interventions is to reduce or occlude the blood flow to hair follicle cells until plasma concentrations of circulating chemotherapy drugs are absorbed or eliminated. Clinical use of ice applications to the scalp before and during chemotherapy administration has not been shown to be effective. Some patients may feel a psychological need to try the ice application regardless of its past failures. The use of both ice and tourniquet techniques have recently been thought to create a tumor cell sanctuary, which may be a great risk in cancers that are widely metastatic, such as leukemia or breast carcinoma.[5]

The possibility of hair loss is devastating for many patients because of the importance of appearance to an individual. Awareness of the psychological impact that loss of scalp and body hair can have on a person and on one's concept of sexuality should guide your initial teaching and follow-up care for the individual.

- Explain alopecia to the patient; emphasize that this side effect is variable and that it is temporary.
- Prepare the patient to expect hair loss two to three weeks after the initial dose.
- Describe cosmetic interventions the patient may use: use of a wig when appropriate; use of scarves or turbans for women.

NAUSEA AND VOMITING

Nausea and vomiting are probably the most frequently encountered side effects of chemotherapy. Symptoms may occur before treatment, shortly after treatment, or be delayed for six to 12 hours and persist for 24 hours or more. Although the incidence of nausea and vomiting may be dose-related with some drugs, the induction and severity of symptoms often depends more on the patient's tolerance and on drug combinations. Multiple causes for nausea and vomiting have been defined in the literature:

- direct gastrointestinal irritation;
- stimulation of the chemoreceptor trigger zone in the medulla oblongata, which is activated by chemicals or toxic substances in the bloodstream;
- a central effect on the vomiting center, a motor and reflex center that coordinates vomiting;
- anticipatory anxiety or association; or
- a combination of all of the above.

According to one study, specific factors that aggravated nausea and vomiting were found to be, in descending order: food or drink, motion or position change, the mention or sight of chemotherapy drugs, and equipment and odors.[6]

USE OF ANTIEMETICS

Patients and nurses seem to agree that antiemetics are helpful. Whether the basis for the patient's response is pharmacological or psychological is unknown and may depend on the individual. The drugs seem to work more effectively when given regularly so that an adequate blood level is maintained.

TABLE 5-2 DRUGS USEFUL IN MANAGEMENT
OF NAUSEA AND VOMITING

Antiemetic	Dose and route	Action site
Compazine (prochlorperazine)	10 mg PO or IM q4h; suppository q6h	Chemoreceptor trigger zone
Inapsine (droperidol)	0.5–1.0 mg IV just prior to chemotherapy and q4h	True vomiting center
Reglan (metoclopramide)	2mg/kg IV just prior to chemotherapy and q2H	Chemoreceptor trigger zone
Tigan (trimethobenzamide)	25mg PO q4–6h; 50–100 mg IM or suppository q8h	Chemoreceptor trigger zone
Torecan (thiethylperazine)	10 mg PO or IM q4h; 10 mg suppository q6h	Chemoreceptor trigger zone
Vistaril (hydroxyzine)	25–50 mg IM just prior to chemotherapy and 25 mg PO q4h	Unknown

Antiemetics can inhibit the effect of drugs on the chemoreceptor trigger zone and depress the true vomiting center. Since side effects are individualized, it is important to evaluate each patient's care individually. Sometimes it takes several cycles of treatment before an effective antiemetic is found. A phenothiazine derivative may control nausea and vomiting for one patient, while a sedative works for another patient. Table 5-2 lists drugs found useful in the management of nausea and vomiting.

Nursing measures used to manage nausea and vomiting include the following:

1. Explain the potential for nausea and vomiting, that it varies patient to patient, and that some patients never experience these symptoms.
2. Instruct the patient to take the antiemetic 30 to 60 minutes prior to treatment to achieve central blocking effect.
3. Encourage the use of antiemetics on a schedule to achieve optimal blood levels.
4. Instruct the patient of potential adverse reactions associated with the antiemetic and to report any side effects.
5. Assess nausea and vomiting status during each visit and re-evaluate antiemetic therapy.
6. Document onset, intensity, and duration of symptoms and response to interventions.

7. Assess dietary habits to help plan foods best tolerated after chemotherapy.
8. Suggest that pretherapy food intake is helpful for some patients.
9. Suggest bland foods that are easy to digest following chemotherapy; urge them to avoid spicy, greasy foods.
10. To improve appetite, appearance, quantity, and quality are factors to consider.
11. Try to keep the environment clean, comfortable, and odor-free. Nausea can be triggered by odors, foods, equipment, sounds, and talking about unpleasant things.
12. Have an emesis basin handy but not in sight.
13. Include family or significant others in care.

STOMATITIS

Stomatitis is a painful and frequent side effect of chemotherapy. About seven days after treatment, the oral mucosa atrophies and thins. This loss of surface mucosa occurs because cell renewal does not keep up with cell destruction. As a result, minor trauma can lead to ulceration and potential infection. Oral mucosa cells and white blood cells have the same renewal rates. About two or three days prior to the white blood cells' lowest point, the oral mucosa begins to deteriorate. This correlation sets the stage for infection. Organisms have an accessible entry, meet no host resistance, and produce infection which may lead to sepsis and possibly death.

Oral mucosa serves as a first line of defense against infection. It initiates digestion, humidifies air, secretes enzymes, lubricates, and facilitates ion exchange. Mucosal cells normally have a life span of 10 to 14 days with continuous replacement. Chemotherapy interferes with cell production, maturation, and replacement. It can also reduce the amount of saliva secreted, resulting in xerostomia.

Those who have had canker sores or burns in the mouth can understand how sensitive and painful stomatitis can be. Stomatitis can interfere with the patient's nutritional status, speech, and ability to rest. For these reasons, prevention and treatment of stomatitis are major nursing concerns.

The following nursing measures can help to prevent stomatitis:

1. Obtain a dental history on the initial visit:

   • presence of full or partial dentures,
   • history of gum disease,
   • usual oral care habits,
   • need for dental work,
   • history of mouth sores, and
   • smoking.

2. Assess the patient's mouth for moisture, color, texture, and debris.
3. Show the patient how to examine the mouth and instruct him to report significant changes.
4. Explain what stomatitis is.
5. Encourage preventive oral hygiene:

   - brush twice daily with soft toothbrush,
   - floss daily,
   - massage gums to stimulate circulation, and
   - cleanse mouth three to four times daily with either baking soda and water (one teaspoon to a cup) or hydrogen peroxide and isotonic saline (made from one teaspoon saline to a quart of water, mixed with equal part of peroxide). Both effectively loosen mucus and crusts but may irritate open sores.

When stomatitis occurs, use the following treatment measures:

1. Frequently assess oral mucosa status.
2. Frequently—three to four times daily—clean the oral cavity with isotonic saline.
3. Hydrate the mouth to maintain adequate lubrication.
4. Use any of various solutions to promote comfort and healing:

   - rinse oral mucosa with 50% Benadryl elixir, 50% Kaopectate four times daily;
   - rinse with viscous Xylocaine (2%) five to 10 minutes prior to eating;
   - rinse with Xylocaine 25 mg, Benadryl 25 mg, and Maalox four times daily; or
   - freeze Xylocaine and favorite juice in 30 ml cups or ice cube tray. Use prn.

Bone Marrow Depression

The bone marrow produces stem cells which mature to become red cells and white blood cells. This continuous process unfortunately is affected by chemotherapy. Not all bone marrow cells are actively dividing all of the time; a significant amount may be in the resting phase. Most chemotherapeutic agents affect only those cells that are actively dividing. Damage to the stem cells or premature blood cells results in a decreased amount of circulating, functional cells.

The absence of blood cells as a result of chemotherapy correlates with the half-life of each cell type. Red cell half-lives are approximately 120 days. Half-lives for platelets and granulocytes, respectively, are five to seven days and six hours. Anemia is usually not apparent, unless aggressive and prolonged treatment is administered. Losses in platelets and granulocyte stem cells rapidly show up in platelet and white blood cell counts. The overall effect of stem cell suppression improves as the production capacity in the recovering stem cell population increases following chemotherapy. It's important when planning patient care to be aware of specific bone marrow suppression nadirs and recovery times associated with each drug.

The following are nursing measures to be used for bone marrow depression:

1. Explain to the patient the significance of the three blood cell types and how chemotherapy can affect them.
2. Stress the purpose and importance of blood counts.
3. Inform the patient that sometimes weekly blood counts are done to monitor the nadir. It's possible that treatment will be postponed if the patient's count is low.

THROMBOCYTOPENIA

4. Explain signs of bleeding the patient should note and report, including bruising; bleeding gums or nostrils; blood in urine, stools, or sputum; and black tarry stools.
5. Encourage safety precautions: no aspirin, only electric razor for shaving.
6. If bleeding, patient should apply steady, firm pressure to site.
7. Instruct the patient to come to the emergency room if bleeding persists.

LEUKOPENIA

8. Explain signs of infection to note and report: elevated temperature, cough, shaking chills, swelling, or redness, and urgency, burning, or frequency of urination.
9. Instruct the patient to stay away from crowds to prevent exposure to contaminants.
10. Encourage the use of sterile or clean technique as appropriate, such as correct hand washing.

ANEMIA

11. Explain signs of a decreased red blood count to note and report: fatigue, pallor, shortness of breath, palpitations, dizziness, chest tightness, and feeling cold easily.
12. Keep in mind that each patient reacts in various ways. You must make assessments and ask questions, because many patients will not report symptoms unless they are specifically asked.

FIGURE 5-1 PATIENT TEACHING RECORD

Area of teaching	Learning content	Initial teaching	Reinforced teaching	Evaluation of learning
Effects of chemotherapy I. Bone Marrow				
A. CBC	1. Purpose of a blood count			
B. WBC	2. Function of white blood cells			
	3. Signs of infection: increased temp/cough, shaking chills, swelling/redness, urgency/burning/frequency of urination			
C. RBC	4. Function of red blood cells			
	5. Signs of decreased red blood cells: fatigue, pallor, shortness of breath			
D. Platelets	6. Function of platelets			
	7. Signs of bleeding: bruising, bleeding of gums/nostrils, blood in urine/stools/sputum, black tarry stools			
E. Patient action	8. Avoidance of aspirin			
	9. Precautions with razors			
	10. Notification of physician or nurse if symptoms of infection, decreased red blood cells, or bleeding occur.			

II. Mucus membranes	1. Signs of stomatitis			
A. Oral cavity	2. Possibility of nausea/vomiting			
B. Stomach	3. Use of antiemetics			
C. Bowel	4. Possibility of diarrhea			
	5. Need for dietary changes			
	6. Use of Kaopectate			
D. Vagina	7. Decreased vaginal secretions			
	8. Possibility of vaginal ulceration			
E. Patient action	9. Notification of physician or nurse if stomatitis, nausea and/or vomiting, or diarrhea persist for more than 24 hours			
III. Hair follicles	1. Possible alopecia			
	2. Use of wig			
IV. Nutritional status	1. Importance of nutrition			
	2. Changes in taste			
	3. Increased protein/carbohydrate diet			
	4. Avoidance of alcohol			
V. Instructional Materials	1. Patient checklist			
A. Drug information	2.			
B. Nutritional materials	3.			
	4.			
	5.			
	6.			

Patient Education

Patient education is an important part of chemotherapy and an important aspect of the nursing process. It prepares the patient and family for the potential desired effects as well as possible side effects of therapy and helps them to determine what to do in the event of a significant change in the patient's body following treatment.

FIGURE 5-2 CHEMOTHERAPY NURSING GUIDELINES,
PATIENT INSTRUCTION

Adriamycin (doxorubicin) an antitumor antibiotic.
Action: Action of this cytotoxic antibiotic is related to its ability to bind to DNA and inhibit nucleic acid synthesis.

Dosage and Preparation: Usual dose range is 30–110 mg every three weeks. Available in 10- or 50-mg vials. Reconstitute with sterile saline (not bacteriostatic water). May be given IV infusion by R.N. or IV push by M.D. Infuse over 15–30 minutes in NS or D5W. Stable 24 hours at room temperature and 48 hours if stored in a refrigerator.

Adverse reactions	Nursing intervention
	Check VS including temperature, before administration.
1. Nausea and vomiting two to six hours after dose.	1. Administer antiemetic as ordered.
2. Total doses over 550 mg/M^2 may cause cardiopathy. This may occur at lower cumulative doses in patient with prior irradiation or on concurrent Cytoxan therapy.	2. Question total dose greater than 550 mg/M^2. Recent EKG should be checked.
3. Urine turns red for up to 12 days after dose.	3. Explain to patient that this is the color of the drug
4. If IV infiltrates local tissue, necrosis will occur.	4. Stay with patient for entire infusion to check for infiltration. If infiltrated, elevate extremity and apply ice immediately for a minimum of eight hours.
5. Rash may occur at site of infusion	5. Wrap extremity with cool towel.
6. Bone marrow depression.	6. Prior to administration, check blood values (CBC, platelets). Notify house staff of abnormal values. Observe for bleeding and signs of infection.
7. Severe alopecia.	7. Scalp tourniquet may be used. Advise patient to purchase a wig ahead of time.
8. Stomatitis.	8. Inspect mouth for sores. Instruct patient in oral hygiene.

Before beginning chemotherapy, develop an individualized teaching plan on the basis of your assessment of the patient's and/or family's learning needs, the treatment schedule, and the home situation. Then present the information, allow time for questions, and provide the patient with written information, including phone numbers of the doctor and nurse available to them (Figures 5-1, 5-2, and 5-3).

Figure 5-1 is a tool to keep in the chart as a teaching guideline and for reinforcement on follow-up visits. Figure 5-2 is an example of a drug information sheet that both you and the patient can use. Figure 5-3 is a checklist that the patient can take home. Most people find it helpful; it's simple and specific about things to do and avoid.

The patient has a responsibility to learn enough about therapy to recognize significant changes and take appropriate action. This is especially important for those on outpatient chemotherapy. Follow-up and evaluation should be ongoing. In some centers, the primary nurse phones the patient following the first treatment to evaluate response, encourage communication, and let the patient know someone is available. The nurse should provide—in writing—the name and phone number of the person who can be called.

Patient instruction

1. Urine may turn orange-red up to 12 days after dose.

2. Nausea and vomiting may occur two to six hours after administration and may last several hours. Take antinausea drug as directed.

3. You may have hair loss 14–21 days later, but this will be temporary. You may wish to wear a wig or toupee until your hair growth resumes. These hairpieces may be covered by your insurance. They are tax-deductible medical expenses.

4. This drug may make you susceptible to infection. Avoid exposure to people who are sick. Use good body and oral hygiene.

5. Notify your doctor if you have: temperature over 100°; chills, cough, sore throat or any other signs of infection; any signs of bleeding (nosebleed, bloody stools, bloody urine, bruising).

6. Check with your doctor before taking any medication, including aspirin, cold remedies, and vitamins.

7. Eat well-balanced meals and check with your doctor before taking alcohol.

8. Examine mouth and gums frequently for sores. If a sore occurs, you may find rinsing mouth with a mixture of one-half hydrogen peroxide and one-half water helpful.

Note: Call your physician if you experience any unusual symptoms or if untoward side effects persist.

FIGURE 5-3 PATIENT INFORMATION CHECKLIST

Diet, nutrition
_____ Take frequent small meals
_____ Eat bland food
_____ Supplement diet
_____ Consult with dietician
_____ Eat banana daily

_____ Drink orange juice daily
_____ Take medications with meals
_____ Take medications fasting
_____ Diet as tolerated

Fluids (intake and output)
_____ Drink fluids one day prior to chemotherapy, day of treatment, and day after. Two to three quarts per day (eight to 12 8-oz. glasses).

_____ Urinate frequently and empty bladder before sleep.

Infection/bleeding caution
_____ Avoid sources of infection.
_____ Call or contact your physician at signs of infection, such as fever, chills, cough, or sore throat.

_____ Do not take aspirin compounds.
_____ Notify physician of any signs of bleeding (skin bruises, black or bloody stools, blood in urine, nose bleeds)

Oral hygiene
_____ Examine mouth and gums frequently; notify your doctor or nurse of any mouth sores.

_____ Use mouthwash
_____ Use soft tooth brush
_____ Keep up regular brushing and dental care.

Drug interactions
_____ Restrict alcohol intake on days of chemotherapy.
_____ Do not take any medication or vitamins unless ordered by the doctor administering chemotherapy.

_____ Use sun screen for any prolonged sun exposure.
_____ Before attempting a permanent wave or hair color, do test strand.

Body hygiene, possible body changes
_____ Bathe as usual.
_____ Tub bath/showers restricted for _____ hours.
_____ Notify your doctor or nurse of change in bowel habits.

_____ Urine orange/red (Adriamycin therapy only)
_____ Prosthesis
_____ Notify your doctor or nurse of any urinary frequency or burning.
_____ Weight gain.
_____ Weight loss.
_____ Purchase wig before hair loss.

Reproductive system

_____ Menstrual irregularities.

_____ Effect on sperm production

_____ Birth control measures

_____ Genital irritation.

Energy conservation

_____ Take frequent rest periods; fatigue is normal.

_____ Insomnia.

_____ Pace activity level according to body needs and chemotherapy cycle.

Care of veins

_____ Use small rubber ball to exercise hand—10 min/day.

_____ Do not use limb on operative side for B/P or venipuncture.

_____ Notify your doctor or nurse of red area or pain around veins.

_____ Veins may take on a darker color.

Sensory

_____ Notify physician of visual or hearing changes, such as ringing in ears, blurring of vision, tearing (eyes may feel like sand is in them).

_____ Notify your doctor or nurse of numbness and tingling of extremities.

Medications

_____ RX for nausea and vomiting

_____ Other medication(s).

_____

_____

_____

_____

_____

This patient information guide cites common possible side effects of chemotherapy and intervention that may minimize the side effects. If you have any other untoward side effects, call your physician.

REFERENCES

1. **Pilapil FS and Studva KV.** Programmed instruction: Cancer chemotherapy. CANCER NURS 1:262, 1978.

2. **Pilapil FS and Studva KV.** Programmed instruction: Cancer chemotherapy—antimetabolites. CANCER NURS 1:340, 1978.

3. **Pilapil FS and Studva KV.** Programmed instruction: Cancer chemotherapy—natural products. CANCER NURS 1:410, 1978.

4. **Zelski LM.** Programmed instruction: Cancer chemotherapy—steroid hormones. CANCER NURS 1:474, 1978.

5. **Dorr RT and Fritz WL.** CANCER CHEMOTHERAPY HANDBOOK. New York: Elsevier, 1980.

6. **Scogna DM and Smalley RV.** Chemotherapy-induced nausea and vomiting. AM J NURS 79:1562, 1979.

BIBLIOGRAPHY

Apple MA. New anticancer drug design: Past and future strategies. In CANCER, A COMPREHENSIVE TREATISE, vol 5, CHEMOTHERAPY, Becker FF (ed). New York: Plenum, 1977.

Cline MJ and Haskell CM. CANCER CHEMOTHERAPY, 3rd ed. Philadelphia: Saunders, 1980.

Daeffler R. Oral hygiene measures for patients with cancer I. CANCER NURS 3:347, 1980.

————. Oral hygiene measures for patients with cancer III. CANCER NURS 4:29, 1981.

Gralla RJ, Itri LM, Pisko SE, et al., Antiemetic efficacy of high-dose metoclopramide: Randomized trials with placebo and prochlorperazine in patients with chemotherapy-induced nausea and vomiting. N ENGL J MED 305:905, 1981.

Krakoff I. Systemic cancer treatment: Cancer chemotherapy. In CLINICAL ONCOLOGY, Horton J and Hill GH (eds). Philadelphia: Saunders, 1977.

Lovejoy NC. Preventing hair loss during Adriamycin therapy. CANCER NURS 2:177, 1979.

Marino LB. CANCER NURSING. St Louis: Mosby, 1981.

Ostchega Y. Preventing and treating cancer chemotherapy oral complications. NURSING 80 10:47, Aug 1980.

Reilly JJ, Neifeld JP, and Rosenberg SA. Clinical course and management of accidental Adriamycin extravasation. CANCER 40:2053, 1977.

Satterwhite B. What to do when Adriamycin infiltrates. NURSING 80 10:37, Feb 1980.

6
RADIATION THERAPY

MICHELLE A. McCLANAHAN, RN, BS

Increased sophistication of machinery, techniques, and knowledge of radiation therapy has resulted in this mode of treatment being used for a large percentage of cancer patients. The goal of radiation treatment is to destroy or significantly alter the tumor mass or radiosensitive cells without serious damage to surrounding normal tissue—in other words, to cure. But radiation therapy is also used when the possibility of cure is remote, to relieve symptoms, prolong life, or relieve pain or obstruction resulting from increasing pressure as the tumor expands.

Radiation treatment is aimed at destroying the tumor cell. Radiosensitivity is greater in cells undergoing mitosis and in those that are oxygenated and that proliferate. Hypoxic cells are more difficult to kill by radiation, as are mature, well-differentiated cells.[1] Certain tissues, such as skin, which has rapid replacement of cells, are more sensitive to radiation than others. The desirable effects of radiation to the tumor mass or cells are cell death, delay of tumor growth, and suppression of motility and reproduction of the cell. As with any mode of treatment aimed at altering the cell structure, abnormal mutations can occur in patients who are in their reproductive years.

Radiation therapy may be the primary form of treatment or it may be used in conjunction with surgery or chemotherapy or both. In this treatment, radiation is focused to a specific body area, and waves of electromagnetic energy result in ionization when they contact body tissues. As the body absorbs this energy, the desired interruption of cellular mitosis occurs.

You have an important role in caring for the patient undergoing radiation treatment. First, you must be familiar with the treatment process and terminology. (Table 6-1 provides a list of commonly used terms.) Second, you must know radiation safety and required precautions. Each hospital that administers radiation treatment should have a radiation safety officer and a manual that provides necessary information about safety precautions.

The Treatment Process

Radiation therapy is a term applied to one mode of treatment for the cancer patient. However, treatment includes more than just the administration of radiation. Radiation treatment starts with the evaluation of each patient. Included in this evaluation are identification of the type of cancer through biopsy, pathology reports, and other measures and determination of the potential susceptibility of the cancer tumor to radiation.

The radiation oncologist formulates a treatment plan for patients selected for radiation treatment. This plan includes the form of administration, required dose, and treatment schedule. The two major forms of delivery of radiation are external and internal. The size, shape, and position of the tumor determine the volume of radiation. The treatment schedule is often referred to as fractionation, which means the delivery of small doses of radiation over a specified period, usually three or four treatments per week for a number of weeks. Fractionation allows the tumor cells to be destroyed while also allowing repair time for the normal cell tissues. Radiation "treatment" includes the care and teaching of the patient before, during, and after treatment.

In some types of cancer, such as skin lesions, the primary approach to treatment may be radiation. In select cases, the patient may have radiation treatments before surgery. This form of combined treatment approach is often used prior to head and neck surgery to improve the resectability of the tumor.[1] Some persons mistakenly believe that radiation is a last resort, but if a patient is not a candidate for surgery, that does not necessarily mean the patient should undergo radiation.

TABLE 6-1 DEFINITION OF TERMS IN RADIATION THERAPY

Curative radiation therapy: treatment whose primary aim is cure.

Dosimeter: small device worn by nursing and radiation personnel to monitor their exposure to radiation while they prov le direct care to patient.

Fractionation: serial small doses of radiation.

Half-life: time it takes for one-half of atoms in a radionuclide to decay or lose one-half of their original energy.

Interstitial radiotherapy: radiation source enclosed in a device (needle, "seed") directly inserted into tumor.

Intracavitary radiotherapy: radiation source inserted into a cavity of the body, such as the intrauterine cavity.

Linear accelerator, betatron, cyclotron: machines that deliver high energy in the administration of radiation therapy.

Port: site of entry of the radiation beam.

Rad (radiation absorbed dose): a unit of measurement of the absorbed radiation dose.

Radiation illness: physical symptoms that are the body's direct reaction to radiation (nausea, vomiting, diarrhea, anorexia, malaise).

Radical radiation therapy: may be primary approach or in conjunction with other forms of therapy (surgery, chemotherapy).

Radionuclide: nucleus of chemical element plus orbiting electrons that have become unstable and emit radiant energy (radioisotope).

Radioresistant: resistant to irradiation; said of tumor cells.

Radiosensitive: susceptible to irradiation; said of tumor cells.

Radium: radioactive material that emits beta particles and gamma rays. When beta particles are shielded by metal, gamma rays can be used in therapy, such as internal implantation.

Rem: (roentgen-equivalent—man): radiation dose that is equivalent in biologic effectiveness to one rad of X-rays.

Roentgen: international unit of measurement of X-rays or gamma rays.

Sealed radioisotope: refers to the radioisotope contained within a specially prepared mold or metal container that is inserted into the patient's body as a temporary or permanent implant.

Unsealed radioisotope: radioisotope that is used either systemically or orally but is not contained within any special container or device.

Postoperative radiation treatment is planned when the tumor has been resected and there is suspicion or proof that residual tumor cells remain either at the surgical site or within the lymph node system. In this event, radiation treatment should follow surgery as soon as adequate wound healing occurs, usually within four weeks. Radiation administered to tissues that have just undergone surgical interruption and are in the process of repair may retard or hinder regrowth or regeneration of tissue. In some cases, this may result in wound infection, increased drainage, or possibly even wound evisceration, dehiscence, or both.[1,2]

In some instances, a surgically resectable tumor—for example, a massive tumor with necrotic cells in its center—may be radioresistant, requiring a higher level of radiation. The surgical procedure itself may interrupt or disperse the tumor cells, thus changing the radiation approach. The potential for spread via the lymphatic system is considered in selection of postoperative radiation treatment.[3]

Radiation treatment may be selected instead of surgical intervention when the malignant lesion cannot be reached through surgery, or when the loss of the organ or organ function that would result from surgery is undesirable.

Patient Teaching

Prior to the start of radiation treatment, patient teaching is a vital physician and nursing responsibility. To adequately prepare the patient, you must know the patient's history, the type of and extent of cancer, the purpose of radiation, the procedure or form of application, and radiation hazards and potential side effects. Assess the patient's level of understanding and anxiety before proceeding with teaching. Information the patient has learned from the physician and those areas the patient does not understand should be clarified. The patient should be made to feel comfortable enough to ask questions.

Pretreatment care may include a tour of the radiation therapy treatment rooms and an opportunity for the patient to meet personnel. During this period of confusion and physical discomfort, it is imperative that all care givers provide the patient with emotional support and an opportunity to express feelings.[4]

The following are practical procedures and considerations you should be aware of.

1. Be sure that the patient has been informed and has consented to the procedure.
2. Each treatment will only last for a few minutes.

3. The treatment process does not hurt.
4. The patient will be scheduled for a specific time for radiation therapy. You should confirm the scheduled time with the radiation department.
5. The mode of transportation—wheelchair or cart—depends on the patient's condition.
6. There may be a short wait in the corridor outside the department, so make sure the hospitalized patient wears slippers and robe.
7. The patient will be brought into the treatment room and positioned on a hard X-ray table. During treatment, those areas that are not to receive radiation will be protected by special shields.
8. The patient will be placed in a specific position, and the X-ray machine will be directed at certain sites on the patient's body.
9. All personnel will leave the room; although the patient will be alone in the room during the treatment, personnel will observe the patient through a window or an intercom system or both.
10. Following completion of the treatment, the patient may be taken from the area with no further care requirements. Patients should be reassured that they are not radioactive and will not endanger family, friends, or hospital personnel.

External Radiation

External radiation is delivered via special megavoltage machines, such as the linear accelerator, betatron, or cyclotron. The development of these high-voltage machines has allowed greater penetration at the desired location with less trauma and damage to surrounding normal tissue and skin. External radiation is a noninvasive procedure. The patient is required to lie on a special table and the beam of the machine is targeted on the area that requires irradiation. A dose, expressed in rads, is formulated according to the area involved, size of the tumor, whether present or recently removed, type of cancer, and the individual patient. The least curable or treatable types of cancer are squamous cell and adenocarcinomas.

NURSING GUIDELINES
Observe the patient for potential side effects during the course of radiation therapy, according to the following guidelines:

1. Frequently observe the skin surface of the radiated area for any redness.

2. If a recent postoperative site is being radiated, check the suture line for:

- increased drainage,
- edges of the wound separating,
- presence or increase of discoloration, and
- increased swelling.

In addition to observation for the occurrence of possible side effects, teach the patient about important precautions. They are:

3. Lotions or cosmetics should not be used in the area where radiation will be targeted, as they may alter the effectiveness of the treatment.
4. The treatment area may be demarcated or outlined with a special ink; patients may lightly wash, but should not remove the markings.
5. Tape should not be used on the patient's skin.
6. Advise the patient to wear comfortable nonrestricting clothing.
7. Extremes in temperature should be avoided.
8. Monitor the patient's fluid and electrolyte balance and nutritional status:

- assess whether the patient is experiencing nausea, vomiting, or dehydration;
- check weight daily;
- regularly monitor laboratory values for electrolytes, BUN, or creatine; and
- promote adequate nutrition; the patient should select appetizing foods and may increase snacks or supplement diet with high-calorie drinks.

9. Evaluation of CBC, blood count differential, and platelets is done to determine the need for blood transfusions. Secondary to the disease process, physical insults of surgery, or other treatments, but especially with radiation, resulting bone marrow depression may require blood transfusions.
10. The patient should be informed of decreased resistance to infections. Teach the patient to be careful to avoid cuts, falls, or contact with persons with contagious diseases, such as colds or viral infections.

If the patient experiences significant side effects, the treatment program may be altered or discontinued. Previously, radiation sickness was a common side effect of radiation treatment. The incidence of radiation sickness has decreased as a result of increased knowledge of radiation administration and improved technology that allows lower doses to be utilized.

Internal Radiation

Internal radiation is administered to patients through implantation, oral ingestion, or systemic administration of radioisotopes, which are either sealed or unsealed.

For appropriate care planning and protection of the patient, yourself, and others, you should know which radioisotope will be used in the treatment of the patient and its half-life, the type of rays the radioisotope emits, and, if unsealed, the route of excretion. In addition to being familiar with the hospital's radiation safety policy, you must know what to do, should items like linen and diet trays become contaminated with the radioactive material.[5]

In some cases, it may be necessary to place the patient in a private room, using isolation precautions for the period of treatment to prevent exposure to others. The patient's room, chart, and Kardex should be properly marked. The patient should know the reason for the isolation. The nurse must use the limited time with the patient efficiently, so that the patient has good physical care and emotional support.

When caring for a patient undergoing internal radiation, remember three basic principles of radiation safety:

- the greater the distance from the source of radiation, the less the exposure;
- the less time in contact with the source, the less exposure; and
- proper shielding from the source, usually of external radiation, is essential to prevent exposure.

Direct patient care should be given efficiently. At all times, wear a dosimeter to monitor your exposure to the radiation.

Throughout the course of radiation treatment, the patient and family need the support of all caregivers. Radiation treatment represents a hope to the patient either for cure or relief of symptoms.

Selected patients with certain types of cancer are treated through the implantation of a radioactive substance or temporary application of it to the part of the body where the carcinoma is located. A radioisotope is "sealed" into a special mold, wire, needle, tube, or applicator. Radioisotopes with a long half-life, such as radium, cobalt-60, cesium-137, are selected for sealed administration.

The two major types of application are interstitial or intracavitary. In interstitial application, special needles are directly inserted into the tumor. Intracavitary application is accomplished by inserting a special mold or application of the radioactive source into a body cavity, such as the cervix or bladder. Intracavitary insertion should be done in the operating room. Once the treatment is complete (usually 24–48 hours), the radioactive implant is removed at the bedside. Shortly after removal, the patient is discharged.

Implants via molds, such as the intracavitary applications, require special care precautions. You should know the site of insertion and monitor bedpans and linen or other items for the presence of the applicator in case it dislodges. Never directly place hands on the radioactive source. A special long metal forceps should be kept at bedside for use if the applicator must be moved. In any case, the radiation therapist should be notified immediately if it becomes dislodged.

Radioisotopes with a short half-life, such as iodine-131 or gold-198, are used in an unsealed form. These are usually administered by oral ingestion or systemic injection. Unsealed radioisotopes expend their energy rapidly and are eventually excreted by the body.

Radioisotopes with a short half-life usually emit gamma rays. They are administered through oral ingestion and the body excretions should be collected in specially marked lead containers. Also, dressings should be disposed of with caution. Patient-care items, such as bedpans and urinals, should be marked. It may be necessary to wear gloves when caring for the patient. Paper or disposable food trays and utensils are used. After the patient is discharged, his room should be thoroughly cleaned.

REFERENCES

1. **DeVita VT, Hellman S, and Rosenberg SA.** CANCER—PRINCIPLES AND PRACTICE OF ONCOLOGY. Philadelphia: Lippincott, 1982.
2. **Khandikar JD and Lawrence GA.** FUNDAMENTALS IN CANCER MANAGEMENT. Niles, Ill: MEL, 1982.
3. **Rubin P.** CLINICAL ONCOLOGY FOR MEDICAL STUDENTS AND PHYSICIANS; A MULTIDISCIPLINARY APPROACH, 6th ed. New York: American Cancer Society, 1983.
4. **Marino LB.** CANCER NURSING. St Louis: Mosby, 1981.
5. **Beyers M and Dudas S.** THE CLINICAL PRACTICE OF MEDICAL-SURGICAL NURSING, 2nd ed. Boston: Little, Brown, 1984.

7

HYPERTHERMIA

KIMBERLY RAIA, RN, MS
JENNIFER COATES, RN, BSN

Over time, hyperthermia has had a variety of meanings. Literally, hyperthermia is an abnormally high temperature. It is sometimes considered synonymous with hyperpyrexia, which means elevated body temperature, but in current usage the term hyperthermia means artificially induced high body temperatures. Hyperthermia was used as a nonspecific agent in the treatment of a variety of conditions, such as inflammatory states and syphilis, in the preantibiotic era.

The treatment of cancer with hyperthermia alone or in combination with a variety of other modalities has a long history. Hyperthermia was attempted prior to Roentgen's discovery of X-rays in 1885. In 1886, Busch described a two-year eradication of facial sarcoma in a patient who had a high fever accompanied by acute localized inflammation. Many authorities, however, regarded this work as unscientific and irresponsible.[1]

In 1893, William Coley described curing advanced cancer in 12 of the 38 patients he treated; these patients developed high fevers secondary to bacterial toxins. He used several toxins, including those from *Streptococcus* and *Serratia,* and developed a product identified as Coley's Toxin. Several other authors reported regression of cancer as a result of high fever or the delivery of heat to the tumor site. Nevertheless, work on hyperthermia continued at a slow pace during the first half of this century. A resurgence of interest in hyperthermia has occurred in the past two decades, due in part to the continuing interest of some researchers but, more importantly, to technological advances in the transmission of heat energy into tumors with more precise control than ever before.

At this stage of technological development in the field of hyperthermia, several modalities of localized heat production are being tried. Intensive investigation is continuing to develop the safest and most effective means of producing local hyperthermia. What is known, however, is that heat does kill tumor cells.

A number of methods can be used to accomplish localized hyperthermia. The techniques most commonly used are radio frequency, microwaves, and ultrasound. Comparison of these methodologies is given in Table 7-1. A brief discussion of each method follows, focusing on the differences in their wave lengths and their frequencies and on the advantages and disadvantages of these techniques.

Radio frequency uses a short wave current approximately 70 feet in length at a frequency of 13.55 MHz. Hertz is the unit of measure for wave frequency. Radio frequency machines produce very large circulating magnetic fields in deep tissue. Currents generated from them within the body produce heat. In the late 1970s, researchers from UCLA developed a radio frequency machine called the Magnetrode which effects both superficial and deep heating.

Radio frequency thus can be used to produce heat in both superficial and deep tissue sites. It allows for nearly uniform heating of all tissues under the heat source, thereby heating both the central and peripheral tissues. Radio frequency, however, cannot be focused on specific tissues within the field of treatment; all tissues appear to be heated. A limiting factor with radio frequency is that it couples or binds more readily to fatty tissue than to muscle, connective tissue, or parenchyma; the current does not effectively penetrate fatty tissue.

Microwaves are the propagation of energy by means of time-varying electric and magnetic fields that give rise to ionic currents; when these currents come in contact with the body, they produce molecular motion within the tissues, which results in heat. Generally, microwaves measure several inches in length, but operate at very high frequencies—approximately 1000 MHz. Deep-tissue heating is possible with this method, but there have been problems with heat penetration and uniformity of heat absorption. Microwaves couple more effectively with connective tissue and parenchyma than with fatty tissue and they can be focused; consequently, selective tissues can be heated. However,

TABLE 7-1 COMPARISON OF LOCALIZED HYPERTHERMIA
METHODOLOGIES

	Radio frequency	Microwave	Ultrasound
Source:	electrical	electrical	mechanical
Wave length	70 feet	inches	thousands of feet
Frequency:	13.56 MHz	1000 MHz	0.2-2 MHz
Heat:	uniform	not uniform	not uniform
Focus:	no	yes	yes

inherent in the use of such high-frequency waves is the hazard of reflected waves to the operator and the environment.

Ultrasound waves are mechanical vibrations. A transducer converts
electrical impulses into mechanical waves. When the transducer is
tightly pressed against the area to be treated, the vibrations cause molecular motion, which results in heat. The waves can be thousands of
feet in length and operate at frequencies of 0.2 to 2 MHz. Ultrasound
waves can penetrate to deep tissues, depending upon the frequencies
used; there is no preferential heating of fatty tissue. The waves can be
focused on specific tissues, but the heat distribution is not quite uniform
throughout the affected area. A limiting factor with this technique is
that ultrasound waves cannot traverse tissue-air interfaces; in other
words, the waves do not penetrate air cavities, such as in the lungs. In
addition, high-density tissues, such as bone and fascia, are known to
absorb the waves.

Biological Basis for Treatment

The exact mechanism of tumor destruction is not well understood. It
is thought that hyperthermia affects tumor cells by:

- causing reduction in protein, RNA, and DNA synthesis;
- producing excessive heat in tissues, which cannot be effectively
  dissipated;
- altering cell membrane permeability;
- activating lysosome systems; and
- sensitizing hypoxic cells.

Most studies of hyperthermia have dealt with the effects of moderate
hyperthermia in the range of 42–44°C (108–111°F), based upon the selective thermal sensitivity of tumor cells over their normal cell coun-

terparts in this temperature range. It seemed at first that this range would be hyperthermia's therapeutic limit, because 45° C (113°F) is the threshold of thermal tolerance for both normal and neoplastic cells. Temperatures above the thermal tolerance cause irreversible critical protein denaturation, which progresses in a linear dose-time relationship. The structural chromosomal proteins, repair enzymes, and membrane components are all denatured by hyperthermia.

Investigators have observed, however, that solid tumors have a relatively poor and physiologically unresponsive blood flow, a finding that suggests that tumors retain more heat than do normal tissues with adaptive vasculature that allow heat dissipation. Researchers, in testing the response of tumor and normal tissues to different ranges of heat, have demonstrated that solid tumors can be heated from 45 to 50°C without injuring normal tissue. Adjacent normal tissue can maintain temperatures well below thermal tolerance, remaining between 42–43°C. Normal tissue responds to heat by blood vessel dilation, which increases blood flow and serves to dissipate the heat. Solid tumors not only heat to higher temperatures than normal tissue, but they also retain their heat longer, since their mechanism for heat release is poor.

The primary effect of hyperthermia appears to be damage to the cell membrane, although the mechanism by which membrane damage causes death is unclear. It is postulated that the lipid composition of tumor cell membrane is disorganized by heat and believed that the altered membrane makes the tumor cell more accessible to certain chemotherapeutic agents.[2]

The normal cell, in response to cellular damage, can activate its lysosomal system and release hydrolytic enzymes, thereby aiding in elimination of cellular debris. Destabilized by heat, particularly heat greater than 43°C, the lysosomal system in tumor cells causes hydrolytic "suicidal" enzymes to be released resulting in tumor cell death.

The presence of hypoxic cells in the tumor core is believed to be the limiting factor for the control of tumor by radiation therapy alone. But when hyperthermia is given in conjunction with radiation to hypoxic cells, the observed response is comparable to that of oxygenatd cells. Thus, it appears that hyperthermia sensitizes hypoxic cells to respond as well as oxygenated cells to radiation.

Effects of Combined Therapies

During the last few years, there has been a growing realization of the synergism between hyperthermia and the other standard forms of cancer treatment—chemotherapy and radiation.

In vitro, a striking synergism in cytotoxicity was observed when hyperthermia (42–43°C) was used in conjunction with certain alkylating agents and certain antibiotics. For example, when thiotepa, an alkylating agent, was combined with hyperthermia, the rate of cell toxicity was found to be approximately linear with increasing temperature. All three nitrosoureas (including BCNU, CCNU, and Methyl-CCNU) and cis-platinum (Cisplatin) have also been observed to have a synergistic effect with hyperthermia. Bleomycin sulfate (Blenoxane) is of particular interest because it was found that bleomycin is synergistic with hyperthermia at temperatures greater than but not below 43°C.[2]

Thus far, CCNU, Methyl-CCNU, fluorouracil (5-FU), cis-platinum, cyclophosphamide (Cytoxan), mitomycin-C, and vinblastine sulfate (Velban) have been used with patients at Evanston Hospital undergoing hyperthermia. All of these drugs have been administered directly before hyperthermia, with the exception of 5-FU, which is administered by intravenous push during the first 10 minutes of hyperthermia.

There is clear evidence that hyperthermia and radiation are synergistic. The degree of synergism is related to heat dose (temperature multiplied by duration), time, and sequence between radiation and hyperthermia. It is known that hyperthermia has its greatest effect on cells in the late S phase of duplication; this is the phase of the cell cycle that is least sensitive to radiation. Thus, there is an apparent rationale for this enhanced effect.

Tumor tissues are poorly oxygenated when compared to normal tissues, and these hypoxic tumor cells are resistant to radiation. However, in the presence of hyperthermia, hypoxic cells respond as well as oxygenated cells to radiation. Unfortunately, normal tissues also have an enhanced response to the combined therapies. Therefore, when using combined therapies, modifications in dosage have to be made. Studies are also being conducted to determine the total effect of the combined use of all three modalities. The sequence of treatment, the length of hyperthermia treatments, and dose modifications of both chemotherapy and radiation therapy are being evaluated.

Implementation and Nursing Care

The machine used for hyperthermia therapy is a radio-frequency device called the Magnetrode (Figure 7-1). It is designed to provide local hyperthermia to any depth without preferential heat absorption in surface tissues. This machine produces radio-frequency electromagnetic waves at 13.56 MHz. The dosage or wattage given to the patient is regulated

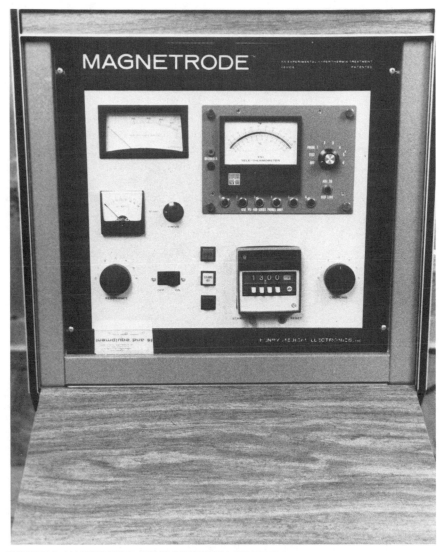

FIGURE 7-1. MACHINE USED FOR HYPERTHERMIA TREATMENT.

by a drive control. A temperature-measurement system is incorporated into the control panel for manual temperature recording during brief periods of treatment cessation. A digital timer is also on the control panel. Coupling and resonance controls are used to bring reflected power or waves to zero. High reflected power results in an increased amount of waves extending beyond the treatment field.

CONTACT ELECTRODES

Tissues with less than one centimeter of overlying subcutaneous tissue may be treated with contact electrodes (Figure 7-2), which are designed for use with water cooling. With these contact electrodes, there is preferential heating of surface and subcutaneous tissues; they cannot be used for heating deep tissues. These electrodes are placed so that they "sandwich" the area that contains the lesion to be heated. In therapy, the electrode that most closely approximates the size of the lesion is selected for use.

For effective therapy, it is essential that the complete electrode is in contact with the skin. The second electrode is placed opposite the first. Because the second electrode most often has complete contact with normal tissue, a water cooling machine is attached to the electrode to cool the tissue and prevent burning.

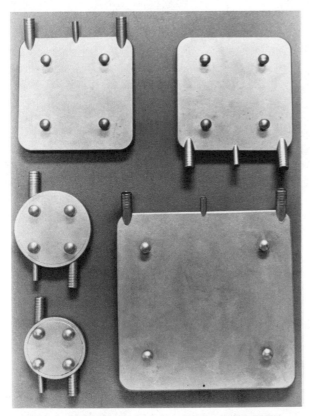

FIGURE 7-2. CONTACT ELECTRODES USED IN HYPERTHERMIA TREATMENT OF SUPERFICIAL OR SUBCUTANEOUS TISSUE.

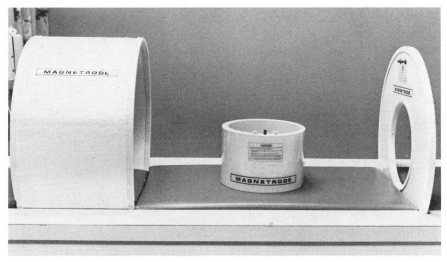

FIGURE 7-3. CIRCUMFERENTIAL NONCONTACT ELECTRODES
USED IN HYPERTHERMIA TREATMENT OF DEEPER TISSUE.

NONCONTACT ELECTRODES

Tissues with greater than one centimeter of overlying surface tissue and deep viscera are treated with circumferential noncontact type electrodes (Figure 7-3). Circumferential electrodes produce very large circulating currents, which induce a strong magnetic field into which the body part is immersed. The heat dosage is determined by a maximum wattage (Table 7-2), which can be safely used with each electrode.

TABLE 7-2 GUIDELINES FOR USE OF CIRCUMFERENTIAL ELECTRODE

Torso pelvis electrode: Accommodates 1000 watts. Start at 700 watts; gradually increase according to tissue temperatures and patient tolerance.

Neck electrode: Accommodates 800 watts. Start at 100 watts; gradually increase according to tissue temperatures and patient tolerance.

Thigh electrode: Accommodates 600–800 watts. Start at 100 watts; gradually increase according to tissue temperatures and patient tolerance.

Precautions:
- When one electrode is in use, the remaining two electrodes *must* be at least five feet away from the one being used.
- Never operate the Magnetrode unless the electrode being used is at least 40 percent filled.

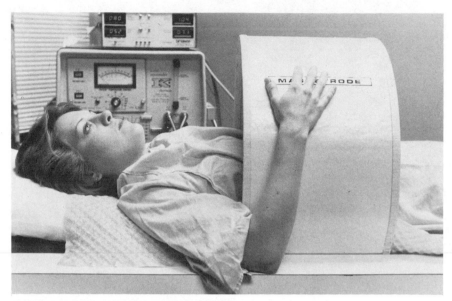

FIGURE 7-4. THE NONCONTACT ELECTRODE FOR
HYPERTHERMIA TREATMENT HEATS BUT DOES NOT GET HOT.
PATIENT MAY TOUCH IT WITHOUT RISKING INJURY.

When using the circular applicators, the treatment area conforms
very closely to the size of the electrode; the waves extend approximately
one to two inches beyond the electrode. These circular electrodes heat
the tissues beneath them, but they themselves don't get hot. Therefore,
a patient can touch the sides of the electrode without fear of injury,
which is particularly comforting if the individual being treated is large
(Figure 7-4).

PATIENT SELECTION
Patients for local hyperthermia are selected by a multidisciplinary team
of physicians representing surgical, radiation, and medical oncology.
Generally, patients who are selected for the program are persons whose
tumors have become resistant to all conventional therapeutic modalities and those persons for whom there is no known effective therapy,
as with carcinoma of the pancreas. It is interesting that investigators
have found no relationship between cell histology and the ability to
be heated. Therefore, a variety of tumor types may be responsive to
this therapy. The sites of tumors treated by hyperthermia at Evanston
Hospital include colorectal, pancreas, lung, melanoma, breast, head and

TABLE 7-3 PROTOCOL FOR PATIENT EVALUATION

1. Patients must be referred to the hyperthermia physicians by a medical doctor.

2. Patient records must be received from the referring physician before an evaluation appointment can be made.

3. Patient records are reviewed by one of the hyperthermia physicians and presented at the group meetings prior to the patient's evaluation appointment.

4. Candidates determined eligible by the group will be examined by the hyperthermia team.

5. Once a patient has been selected and has agreed to begin hyperthermia, the patient's primary physician, if other than one of the hyperthermia physicians, is contacted should the patient experience problems not directly relating to hyperthermia.

neck, esophagus, connective tissue, skin, ovarian, mesothelial, renal, bladder, gastric, and appendiceal.

Initially, the hyperthermia team evaluates the patient's medical record to determine if the patient is an acceptable candidate. The protocol used for this evaluation is shown in Table 7-3. The record is reviewed for extent of disease, tissue confirmation of malignancy, and treatments received. The patient is then examined by the medical team. Particular attention is paid to the site and extent of disease, the ability to measure disease response, and the nutritional and physical status of the patient. Individuals must not be in bed more than 50 percent of the time to be eligible. Experience has shown that people who are ambulatory at least 50 percent of the time tolerate treatments better and are better able to complete the recommended treatments.

An initial evaluation meeting is held, and the patient is given a copy of the specific consent form outlining the investigative nature of the treatment. The patient is also given an opportunity to express concerns and ask questions. The nurse is an important member of the team and often remains with patients and helps them to formulate questions and assists in clarifying their feelings. Since this type of treatment is so new, many people may need help in thinking through the implications of treatment.

IMPLEMENTATION OF THERAPY

Once a patient's eligibility has been established and the patient has consented to treatment, a series of laboratory tests is required. The laboratory protocol used is shown in Table 7-4. In addition, tumor

TABLE 7-4 PROTOCOL FOR LABORATORY EVALUATION

1. Each new patient selected for hyperthermia therapy requires blood tests, including CBC, differential, platelets, SMA-C. Tests are done
   - before and after the first cycle of therapy and
   - before each subsequent cycle of hyperthermia therapy.

2. Patients who have primary or secondary liver involvement require a PT and PTT in addition to the above blood tests.

3. Patients who will receive hyperthermia treatments over the chest area must have an ECG and chest X-ray prior to therapy.

4. Some patients will need coagulation studies completed prior to and during hyperthermia.

TABLE 7-5 INITIAL TREATMENT PROTOCOL

1. A physician from the hyperthermia team must be present during the patient's initial treatment.

2. The physician is responsible for obtaining the patient's signed consent form.

3. During the initial treatment, the physician will determine the electrode field, wattage range, patient tolerance, and safe vital sign parameters.

4. The nurse takes temperature measurements during the initial treatment.

5. For subsequent treatments, the physician from hyperthermia team will prescribe the appropriate wattage range. The nurse may lower, but not raise the wattage, based on patient tolerance.

TABLE 7-6 TISSUE TEMPERATURE PROTOCOL

1. Skin and subcutaneous temperature measurements must be taken on day 1 of cycle 1 for all patients entering the hyperthermia protocol. Tumor temperature should also be taken when possible.

2. Subsequent temperature measurements must be done at least weekly.

3. Wattage limits depend on subcutaneous temperatures and patient tolerance. Therefore, wattage should not be raised unless temperatures are being measured.

4. Ideal subcutaneous temperature range is between 42.5 and 43°C for the "actual," not the observed, readings.

measurements are taken prior to each treatment series to determine treatment effectiveness. If the tumor cannot be physically measured, a CT scan is required. Repeat scans will be subsequently taken to evaluate treatment effectiveness.

TEMPERATURE MEASUREMENT

During the first hyperthermia treatment, a physician from the team must be present. The initial treatment protocol is shown in Table 7-5. Temperatures of the subcutaneous tissue in the treatment field and, when possible, in the tumor are measured. The subcutaneous temperature must not exceed 43°C. The tissue temperature protocol is shown in Table 7-6.

A computerized multichannel thermometry system is utilized to document temperature changes in both tumor and normal tissues. This system allows for constant temperature readings throughout the hyperthermia treatment. It is nonmetallic and, consequently, does not conduct heat when left within the field of treatment. Using sterile technique, the physician implants a 16-gauge Jelco needle into the tissue to be measured. A smaller closed-end sterile tube is passed through the Jelco and left in place throughout the treatment. The thermometer is passed through this closed sterile system, eliminating the need to sterilize the thermometer after each patient. The thermometer is an extremely delicate instrument and can be easily damaged if mishandled. When possible, the closed-end sterile tube is surgically implanted into tumor tissue. It remains in place while the patient undergoes treatment, allowing temperature monitoring to document effectiveness.

It can be expected that equipment used for hyperthermia will be improved as new technology is developed.

SELECTION OF OPTIMAL TEMPERATURE RANGE

Temperatures are taken prior to treatment to establish a baseline. For each patient, temperatures must be taken initially to determine the power per time and dose that will result in optimal temperature range, 42.5–43°C for subcutaneous tissue. Once the optimal temperature is determined in each patient, one can predict temperatures in a specific patient if the treatment variables of *dose* and *time* are constant. Tumor heating and dose and time effects cannot yet be predicted in a new patient without first monitoring tissue temperatures.

A physician must be present for each initial treatment to take tissue measurements and to identify dose and time intervals. Thereafter, the nurse remains with the patient to monitor tolerance and responses. Tolerance parameters—shown in Table 7-7—have been established to guide the nurse in the administration of the treatment.

TABLE 7-7 TOLERANCE PARAMETERS

---

1. Hyperthermia should be stopped and the physician notified when the patient's
   - pulse increases to greater than 135/min;
   - systolic blood pressure reaches 180 mmHg; or
   - diastolic blood pressure reaches 110 mmHg.

2. The physician may specify lower or higher parameters, depending upon the patient's medical limitations.

3. The patient's level of comfort should be assessed at each treatment interval (1 = comfort; 10 = extreme discomfort). When a patient's discomfort reaches 10, the treatment should be discontinued for a period of one or two minutes.

4. Treatment interruptions due to variations in vital signs and patient discomfort should not exceed two minutes. If additional time is required more than once in a treatment period, the physician must be notified and treatment stopped for that day.

5. Treatment intervals are to be between 10 and 20 minutes long. If patients cannot tolerate this interval because of discomfort or vital sign deviations;
   - the treatment should be stopped;
   - the physician is notified; and
   - referral is made for relaxation guidance.

THE TREATMENT PROCEDURE

The patient lies on an ice mattress, on top of a table, which is used to aid in cooling. Baseline oral temperature, pulse, respirations, and blood pressure are taken before the treatment begins. During the treatment, the pulse and blood pressure are constantly monitored by an electronic sphygmomanometer.

Treatments are usually given at 10- to 15-minute intervals, with one- to two-minute rest periods in between. The treatment goal is to give the patient 30 to 60 minutes of hyperthermia. The nursing challenge is to aid the patient in reaching the 30 to 60 minutes with as little physical and psychologic discomfort as possible.

During the treatment, the patient generally experiences feelings of intense heat, described as similar to being in the sun too long or having an extended sauna. Cool cloths are placed on the brow, chest, and often the abdomen to aid in cooling; the patient is also offered sips of cold water. Some individuals also experience a burning sensation in the sternum or coccyx when the treatment area covers the chest or pelvic areas. It is not clear why this occurs. One theory is that these large bones act as antennae to attract the heat. The patient's discomfort begins to decrease as soon as the heat is turned off. Other patients report having this burning sensation in areas of scar formation due to previous surgery and in areas where gross tumor or ascites is present. Cold cloths or ice packs applied to the area are often beneficial.

In addition to the application of cold cloths, patient discomfort may be relieved by use of analgesics, diversion, or other means. Oral acetaminophen with codeine, oxycodone (Percodan), or intramuscular meperidine (Demerol) 30 minutes to one hour prior to the treatment, has relieved discomfort for some patients. Other individuals who experience discomfort are aided by diversional conversation or listening to music, whether it is on the radio or their favorite tape cassette. The nurse may also refer the patient to the department of psychiatry for assistance in learning relaxation aids or self-hypnosis.

Side Effects

Side effects that have been observed during hyperthermia treatment include skin burns, fat necrosis, vital sign variations, and dehydration.

BURNS

Superficial second-degree skin burns have been noted on pressure points, in skin-grafted areas, and where skin touches skin. Burns from the former two cannot be prevented, but the nurse must assess the occurrence of inflammation and minor burns must be assessed and treated appropriately. Thus far, minor burns have occurred in only one percent of patients receiving therapy in Evanston Hospital.

When contact electrodes are used, mild burns are expected over the tumor and in immediately adjacent normal tissue. When minor burns occur, they are kept clean and dry; no additional care has been required. Treatments are continued unless the burns become severe.

Areas where skin has been grafted are more susceptible to burning, as the vascular supply is poor and the mechanism for heat release is inadequate. In the process of attempting to sterilize the tumor, the skin graft may need to be replaced.

The minor burns that can result from skin touching skin can easily be alleviated by placing cloths between the areas touching. For example, cloths can be packed in the axilla and between the arm and the torso; cloths should also be placed under the breasts.

FAT NECROSIS

Thus far, necrosis in subcutaneous fat has been observed in one patient at Evanston Hospital. Necrosis appeared in the upper arm and bilaterally in the breasts; the treatment field was the lungs. Ice packs applied immediately after treatment may decrease the extent of necrosis. Analgesics are given for discomfort. Patients are monitored for signs of infection. If an abscess occurs, it is drained. When patients with fat necrosis are continued on treatments, the temperature in the area of necrosis should not exceed 42.5°C.

CARDIOVASCULAR PROBLEMS

Hyperthermia therapy may initiate excessive increases in pulse and blood pressure that indicate undue strain on the cardiovascular system. Variations in pulse and blood pressure are expected during treatments (see Table 7-7) as indications of the normal cardiovascular response that enables the body to cool itself, thus keeping the core body temperature within a safe range.

Action must be initiated if the patient's acceptable vital-sign range is exceeded twice, even after allowing a two-minute break from treatment. The physician is notified, and treatment is stopped for the day. If the vital-sign range is consistently above the acceptable range, medication such as propanolol or digoxin may be prescribed by the physician. The patient may be released from treatment if medication does not effectively control the pulse and blood pressure. Treatment is not given if the patient's pulse is below 50 or the blood pressure is below 90/50 mm Hg, due to possible vasodilatation, which may occur secondary to the heat.

DEHYDRATION

The most serious problem resulting from hyperthermia therapy can be dehydration. Patients lose excessive amounts of fluid through profuse perspiration and increased respirations. Patients are encouraged to consume at least two liters of fluid per day. A complete blood chemistry and hematocrit and hemoglobin must be obtained before the initial treatment cycle begins to establish baseline data and before each subsequent cycle of treatment to monitor for changes in status.

Dehydration occurs either because there is a decrease in water relative to sodium or a water deficiency. The patient must be monitored for signs and symptoms of dehydration.

NUTRITIONAL DEFICIENCY

Nutritional status is also closely assessed in patients receiving hyperthermia, and may indicate dehydration due to a decrease in fluid intake. The patient who undergoes multiple treatments needs adequate nutrition to assist the body in recovering from cellular breakdown from the combined therapies. Patients who have lost more than 20 pounds before therapy begins are referred to a dietician for consultation and need continuous monitoring for a change in weight, anorexia, and a change in the nutritional status.

EMOTIONAL RESPONSES

Psychosocial support during therapy is of extreme importance. The multiple therapies can be very strenuous for a patient who may already be in a weakened state. People who undergo hyperthermia must also cope with the knowledge that their disease has responded poorly to conventional therapies and that hyperthermia may be their last hope. The hyperthermia nurse is with the patient for at least 40 minutes several times a week and has an opportunity to assess his or her emotional status. The nurse creates an environment in which the patient feels free to discuss problems and concerns and to express feelings. Open-ended sentences can be useful in helping the patient verbalize.

It has been observed that if patients are anxious they seem to tolerate the treatment poorly. If an effective, trusting rapport can be established between patient and nurse, the treatments seem to go faster for the patient and cause less physical and emotional discomfort. If a patient is assessed as being unable to effectively cope with the treatment, a psychologist should evaluate the situation.

INTOLERANCE TO THERAPY

Unfortunately, not all patients can tolerate hyperthermia in spite of interventions and referrals. Consequently, hyperthermia termination guidelines have been established. A patient becomes ineligible for continuing hyperthermia treatments if:

1. Treatment intervals are consistently less than 10 minutes due to patient discomfort or uncontrolled vital-sign elevations.
2. Time between treatment intervals is consistently greater than two minutes due to patient discomfort or vital-sign elevations.
3. Tumor temperatures do not reach the therapeutic range.

In the experimental program at Evanston Hospital, treatments have been terminated for the following reasons:

- disease progression,
- pain,
- discomfort,
- cardiovascular problems, and
- problems unrelated to cancer.

When treatment is terminated, care is taken to ensure that all the patient's hope is not stripped away. Continued contact with at least one of the physicians on the hyperthermia team and the nurse is essential.

The effectiveness of localized hyperthermia has to be further evaluated. Some encouraging results have been observed. But experimentation with regard to treatment scheduling, length of treatment, and dose modification is continuing.

REFERENCES

1. **Pilawal B.** CONCEPTS IN HYPERTHERMIA, doctoral dissertation. Madison, Wis: University of Wisconsin, 1979.
2. **Scanlon, EF.** HYPERTHERMIA GRANT PROPOSAL. Evanston, Ill: Evanston Hospital, 1981.

BIBLIOGRAPHY

Hall EJ. RADIOBIOLOGY FOR THE RADIOLOGIST, 2nd ed. New York: Harper & Row, 1978.

MAGNETRODE: AN EXPERIMENTAL HYPERTHERMIA TREATMENT DEVICE FOR INVESTIGATIONAL, RESEARCH, AND HEAT THERAPY, brochure 80-HME01. Los Angeles: Henry Medical Electronics.

Scanlon EF. HYPERTHERMIA. Evanston, Ill: Evanston Hospital, 1980.

Storm FK, Harrison WH, Elliot RS, et al. Normal tissue and solid tumor effects of hyperthermia in animal models and clinical trials. CANCER RES 39:2245, 1979.

————. Hyperthermic therapy for human neoplasms: Thermal death time. CANCER 46:1849, 1980.

8
IMMUNOTHERAPY

MARY E. MIELNICKI, RN, BSN

Immunotherapy is a relatively new treatment mode and is in experimental stages. Lower animals have been successfully immunized by a variety of techniques. In them, the development of carcinogens and virus-induced tumors have been prevented, and some established tumors have been reduced. As a result of these experiments, immunotherapy has been applied in treatment of oncology patients, and experimentation in this treatment continues, aided by improved technology and increased knowledge about the immune system.

Oncological immunotherapy is based on knowledge of principles of the natural immune process. The normal immune response is triggered whenever an invading organism or protein is present. The invading organism or protein is called an antigen. An antibody is a soluble protein that defends the body against antigens. How does the body discriminate its own proteins from foreign protein bodies? The self-marker theory provides an answer to this question. According to the theory, the body's own proteins have definite molecular structures unique to its own cells. Therefore, antibodies are produced when a protein body with a different molecular structure is recognized.

The immune response can be triggered in several ways. Natural immunity is the resistance against infection that an individual inherits genetically. Acquired immunity—also called active immunity—is the development of antibodies in the body in response to bacteria or viruses. Passive immunity is effected by the introduction of acquired antibodies from other human sources into the body. In cancer immunotherapy, the immune response can be stimulated by nonspecific immunotherapy or it can be specifically directed to the tumor by the introduction of vaccine (active) or by the introduction of tumor antibodies from an immune person. There is the risk of rejection of antibodies acquired from other human sources. Research on immunotherapy in tumor cells is based on the following:

1. The immune system can kill tumor cells by zero kinetics. This means that the immune system works on a fixed number of cells. Because of this, immunotherapy could be curative.
2. In the tumor cell, both the cell membranes and the cell body contain antigens.

Types of Immunotherapy

Four basic types of immunotherapy are being studied in current therapy. They are active immunization, nonspecific stimulation, passive immunization, and adoptive immunotherapy. Each type is described briefly below.

ACTIVE IMMUNIZATION
Antigens, cells from either the patient or a patient with a like tumor, introduced into the body of the patient, stimulate the production of specific antibodies. Antigens can be obtained from inactive cells that were treated and frozen or irradiated.

NONSPECIFIC STIMULATION
There are many nonspecific therapies that stimulate a general immune response. Some of these are:

- BCG (bacille Calmette-Guerin),
- C-Parva (*Corpebacterium parvum*),
- MER (methanol extracted residue), and
- chemicals such as DNCB (dinitrochlorobenzene).

BCG is the most widely used in immunotherapy. The vaccine is usually applied by a scarring technique, but it can be directly injected into the tumor site. BCG is most commonly used to treat acute lymphocytic and myelocytic leukemia as well as malignant melanoma. Side effects of BCG include painful or pruritic areas in or around test site, localized abscess, ulceration, fever and chills, and malaise. Side effects from intralesional injection are hyperpyrexia, hypotension, convulsions, and dusky skin color. Other side effects are adenitis; itching, scaling, or festering of the skin; jaundice (usually temporary); and elevated SGOT and/or alkaline phosphatase.

Interferon is an active, nonspecific immune treatment whose effectiveness is being evaluated. The mechanism of interferon's action is not clear. Interferon works by activating "killer cells" as well as directly damaging tumor cells. Natural interferon from leukocytes is given IM daily in many different strengths over various lengths of time. Interferon is being studied for the treatment of most types of cancer, but no definite results are yet available.

There are many known side effects and adverse complications of interferon therapy. These include vomiting, nausea, fever, chills, headache, fatigue, anorexia, alopecia, weight loss, granulocytopenia, thrombocytopenia, abnormalities of liver enzymes, abnormal cardiac rhythms, and hypotension.

Because of the severe side effects and the fact that it is given daily for a long period of time, patient's tolerance level may decrease, thus diminishing the value of interferon as a treatment for cancer.

PASSIVE IMMUNIZATION

Passive immunization therapy is the direct transfer of cells from persons with established immunity to the tumor cells. Examples of this kind of treatment are: plasmapheresis, lymphocytic therapy, and bone marrow transplant.

Bone marrow transplant is the most common passive therapy performed with significant results. About one-third of patients with bone marrow transplants survive a year following the procedure. Matched bone marrow from a donor, usually a relative, is transplanted to the patient after massive doses of radiation and chemotherapy have been administered to leukemic cells in the patient's bone marrow. During this treatment, the patient is placed in a sterile room and is given massive doses of antibiotic therapy to "sterilize" the intestinal tract.

Marrow transplants are done in highly specialized care centers. The exact precautions and procedures vary. You can help patients develop a general understanding of the treatment and should inform them of the risks of bone marrow transplantation.

The patient's body may reject the graft or bone marrow transplantation. Rejection rarely occurs if proper immunosuppression is done. One possible serious complication of bone marrow transplantation is the graft versus host reaction. Lymphocytes from the donor's bone marrow release lymphokines that injure and kill host cells by direct contact. They attack the skin first, then the intestines and liver.

ADOPTIVE IMMUNOTHERAPY

Adoptive immunotherapy is the introduction of cells or cell products that are tumor-immune into the tumor-bearing patient.

Immunotherapy is still an experimental therapy for oncology patients. Nursing assessment is of major importance in caring for these patients. Observing for allergic reactions, signs of infection, and general changes in the patient is essential.

BIBLIOGRAPHY

Krol MA. The patient with cancer. In THE CLINICAL PRACTICE OF MEDICAL-SURGICAL NURSING, 2nd ed., Beyers M and Dudas S. Boston: Little, Brown, 1984.

McKhann C. Cancer immunotherapy: A realistic appraisal. CA 30:286, 1980.

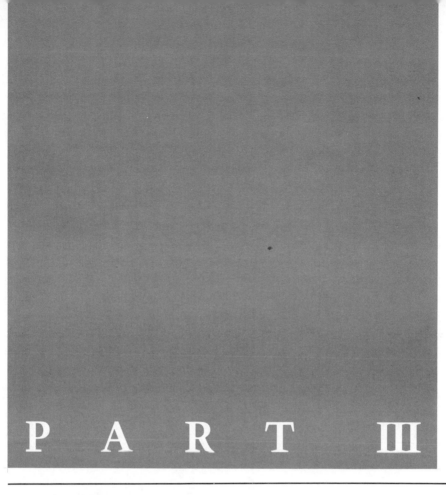

PART III

NURSING MANAGEMENT OF LONG-TERM CARE

9

BLOOD COMPONENT THERAPY

MARY E. MIELNICKI, RN, BSN

The nursing role in caring for patients receiving blood component therapy includes preparing the patient for transfusions, providing the patient with information about the procedure and purpose of the therapy, ensuring safe administration of transfusions, making the patient as comfortable as possible during the transfusion, assessing the patient for the occurrence of side effects or transfusion reactions, and taking appropriate action if reactions do occur.

Indications for Use

Blood component therapy is indicated when the cancer patient is anemic, thrombocytopenic, or leukopenic. These states often result from chemotherapy or are part of the disease process. Thus blood component therapy is a common aspect of chronic cancer. Each of these states is described below.

ANEMIA

Anemia, by definition, is reduction in the number of red blood cells, amount of hemoglobin, and volume of packed red blood cells per 100 ml blood. In the cancer patient, anemia can be caused directly by the disease process, as in a metastatic bone tumor that displaces the marrow of the cavity. Chemotherapy agents can also decrease the production of blood components or destroy stem cells and cause drug-induced anemia. Thrombocytopenia resulting from chemotherapy can cause direct bleeding that leads to anemia. Chronic illness can also result in depressed red cell production. The cause is unknown, but one theory is that erythropoietin production is decreased by the overall deterioration of the patient's physical status.

Normal hemoglobin levels range from 12 to 16 gm. A hemoglobin level above 10 gm is acceptable. Low hemoglobin levels are usually accompanied by signs and symptoms of anemia. They include shortness of breath, dyspnea, pallor of skin and nailbeds, weakness, and vertigo.

Treatment of anemia in the cancer patient begins with identification of the cause. Usually no treatment is immediately indicated if the patient is:

- asymptomatic,
- not actively bleeding, or
- evidencing effects of decreased red cell production as a result of current treatment, and the production is expected to increase soon.

When treatment is indicated, transfusions are administered to decrease the severity of the patient's symptoms. Used for this purpose, transfusions are supportive therapy. In administering transfusions of whole blood and red cells, normal saline is also used with a Y tubing. The transfusion is usually administered over a period of two to four hours. Rate of flow depends on the patient's cardiac history and general physical condition.

THROMBOCYTOPENIA

Platelets circulate in the body at a normal concentration of 150,000 to 350,000 per cubic millimeter. They perform three important functions in blood clotting:

- they adhere to the wall of an injured vessel, which is the first step in coagulation;
- they release incomplete thromboplastin, which aids in the formation of a permanent clot; and
- they release a protein that has the ability to contract and shrink the clot.

Thrombocytopenia is a decrease in platelets that can be caused by decreased production or increased destruction of platelets. Acute leukemia is an example of a bone marrow replacement problem that can lead to thrombocytopenia. The immature granulocyte increases in volume in the marrow, destroying platelet cells and also decreasing the production of all the blood cells in the marrow. Patients with a platelet count of 100,000 per cubic millimeter are at risk. Signs of thrombocytopenia are excessive bleeding, bruising, bleeding of gums, blood in urine, and black tarry stools.

Treatment of thrombocytopenia depends on the patient's condition. Platelets are given commonly in myelosuppressed patients at a rate of six to 10 units at intervals of three to seven days. In cancer patients, platelets are not given unless the patient is symptomatic. Single-donor platelets are preferred to random-donor platelets. Random-donor platelets are usually pushed and must be given soon after they are prepared. Single-donor platelets can be hung over a period of 30 to 60 minutes because they are more stable than random-donor platelets.

LEUKOPENIA

Leukocytes are the white blood cells in the body. Two major types of leukocytes are polymorphonuclear leukocytes and mononuclear leukocytes. Polymorphonuclear leukocytes include neutrophils, eosinophils, and basophils, which are granular in appearance and myelogenous, that is, formed in the bone marrow. Mononuclear leukocytes are the lymphocytes and monocytes. Both are formed mainly in the lymph nodes and lymph tissues. The main function of lymphocytes is to release antibodies against antigens in the body. Monocytes are the second line of defense in fighting infection. Leukocytes live about 14 hours in the bloodstream. If the patient has an active infection, they live only one to two hours.

Leukopenia is the decrease of the white blood cells in the blood. The normal white cell count is 6,000 to 9,000 per cubic millimeter. In the cancer patient, the main cause of leukopenia is myelosuppression as a result of chemotherapy, but it also can result from tumor growth in the bone marrow, which may decrease production of white cells. Granulocytic leukemia also decreases production of mature leukocytes in the blood.

Signs of leukopenia are not as apparent as those of thrombocytopenia and anemia. Signs of infection, such as chills, fever, and sinusitis, may indicate a decrease in leukocytes. A white cell count of 3,000 per cubic millimeter is a caution sign for the cancer patient.

Patients with leukopenia are taught to avoid infections. Treatment consists of antibiotic therapy if indicated. Granulocytes are prescribed infrequently and most commonly to patients with granulocytic leukemia. The criteria for giving granulocyte therapy are:

- fever lasting longer than 48 hours;
- patient on antibiotic therapy for more than 24 hours;
- negative blood cultures;
- granulocyte count less than 500; and
- patient in shock.

Granulocytes are transfused with a Y tubing and isotonic solution to minimize cell lysis. A microaggregate filter should not be used, as it interferes with platelet infusion that may be mixed in suspension. Granulocytes are given over a two- to four-hour period. Vital signs should be taken 15 minutes after the transfusion is begun and every half-hour for two hours, and then at the one-hour intervals until the transfusion is completed.

Patients often have fever and chills when being transfused with granulocytes. The cause of this febrile response is not known. Transfusions are not stopped when fever occurs, but the physician should be notified. The rate of transfusion can be slowed to four hours to decrease symptoms. Acetaminophen and comfort measures are used to help the patient relax. Other signs of a reaction such as hives, rash, wheezing, or hypotension along with a fever indicate that the infusion should be stopped and a physician called immediately.

Granulocytes have a short intravascular survival time and, therefore, are usually administered daily until the patient's own granulocytes increase or the infection is under control.

Administration of Blood Component Therapy

Patients may find blood transfusions more frightening than chemotherapy or radiation treatment. Lack of knowledge about blood therapy, the purpose of therapy, the source of blood, side effects of transfusions, and the meaning of blood therapy as an indication of progression of the disease all contribute to the patient's emotional response. Blood therapy may require hospital admission. The occurrence of leukopenia, thrombocytopenia, and anemia may indicate to them that their disease is progressing and that initial treatment was not effective. By providing clear, factual information about the therapy and the patient's condition you can help the patient cope with anxiety. Listening to the patient and family concerns and answering questions honestly also help decrease the patient's anxiety. *Continued on page 196.*

TABLE 9-1 TRANSFUSION REACTIONS

Hemolytic reaction

Cause:	Administration of mismatched blood.
Pathology:	Antibodies from the patient react with antigens from the donor's blood cell, causing the donor cell to clump. The clumping obstructs blood flow, which, if continued, leads to vital-organ damage, such as renal failure.
Symptoms:	Oliguria, headache, dyspnea, chills, fever.
Treatment:	Push dextrose IV fluid to counteract shock and promote diuresis. Administer oxygen and epinephrine for respiratory complications. If oliguria occurs, insert an indwelling catheter, administer diuretics as ordered by the physician.
Nursing actions:	• Stop blood. • Notify physician. • Check vital signs every 15–30 minutes until stable. • Measure and record intake and output precisely. • Treat as ordered by physician.

Bacterial transfusion reaction

Cause:	Administration of contaminated blood.
Pathology:	Septicemia causing shock. Bacterial reaction can cause "red shock," characterized by flushing of the skin, as differentiated from the paleness of septic shock.
Symptoms:	Vasodilation evidenced by flushed skin, chills, headache, diarrhea, fever.
Treatment:	Push dextrose fluid. Administer vasopressor drugs, corticosteroids, broad-spectrum antibiotics as prescribed by the physician.
Nursing actions:	• Stop blood. • Notify physician. • Check vital signs every 15–30 minutes until stable. • Measure and record intake and output precisely. • Treat as ordered by physician.

Allergic reaction

Cause:	Exact cause unknown. Possibly caused by drug or food byproduct in donor's blood.
Pathology:	Mild reaction—hives, bronchial wheezing, mild edema; *severe reaction*—bronchial spasms, acute respiratory distress.
Treatment:	Administer antihistamines, antipyretics, vasopressors, epinephrine respiratory therapy as prescribed by the physician.
Nursing actions:	• For mild reactions, slow rate of transfusion; notify physician. • For severe reactions, stop blood; notify physician.

Circulatory overload

Cause:	Too rapid infusion of fluid, blood, or normal saline. Elderly patients and those with history of chronic heart failure are at greatest risk.
Pathology:	Acute pulmonary edema, heart failure (left side).
Symptoms:	Tachycardia, hypertension, edema, dyspnea.
Treatment:	Treat with digitalis for chronic heart failure, as prescribed by the physician.
Nursing actions:	• Stop blood and slow normal saline to keep open. • Notify physician. • Check and record vital signs every 15 minutes. • Treat as ordered by physician.

ADMINISTRATION OF BLOOD

Prepare patients by informing them of the purpose of the transfusion and explain the procedure. Give patients time to prepare for the transfusion so that they can rest comfortably during it. You'll promote the patients' rest if you tell them approximately how long the transfusion will take as well as what restrictions the therapy imposes on activity. Make patients as comfortable as possible, giving pain medication as necessary, helping them to comfortable positions, and providing diversion such as television viewing.

There are certain precautions that must be followed for safe blood transfusions:

1. All blood should be checked to ensure that the label on the bag matches the recorded information on the patient's chart for:

   • name, room number, and hospital number.
   • blood type, crossmatch, and special typing factors such as Rh.
2. The name on the label on the bag should match the name on the patient's arm identification band.
3. The patient's vital signs are checked and recorded before hanging the blood. These baseline data are used for evaluating further vital signs. Vital signs are checked 30 minutes after the infusion is started and every 30 minutes until completed.
4. The rate of infusion, as ordered by the physician, is determined by the patient's medical history and physical status at the time of infusion. Ensure that the desired rate is maintained.
5. The patient should be assessed for signs of blood reactions as described below.

TRANSFUSION REACTIONS

Observe the patient for blood transfusion reactions and for signs of circulatory overload when you check vital signs. Patients should also be asked to call the nurse if they notice any unusual signs or symptoms during the transfusion.

The major types of reactions are hemolytic, bacterial, and allergic. They are described in Table 9-1, page 194.

BIBLIOGRAPHY

Baldonado AA and Stahl DA. CANCER NURSING, A HOLISTIC MULTIDISCIPLINARY APPROACH, 2nd ed. New Hyde Park, NY: Medical Examination, 1982.

Graham V and Rubal BJ. Recipient and donor response to granulocyte transfusion and leukophoresis. CANCER NURS 3:97, 1980.

Hernandez B. Platelets: A short course. RN 43:37, June 1980.

Isler C Newest treatment for cancer: Immunotherapy. RN 39:35, April 1976.

———. Newest treatment for cancer: Immunotherapy. RN 39:29, May 1976.

Luckmann J and Sorensen KC. Blood transfusions and reactions. In MEDICAL-SURGICAL NURSING; A PSYCHOPHYSIOLOGIC APPROACH, 2nd ed. Philadelphia: Saunders, 1980.

Patterson P. Granulocyte transfusion: Nursing considerations. CANCER NURS 3:101, 1980.

Price S and Wilson L. PATHOPHYSIOLOGY: CLINICAL CONCEPTS OF DISEASE PROCESSES. New York: McGraw-Hill, 1978.

Walker P. Bone marrow transplant: Second chance for life. NURSING 77 7:24, Jan 1977.

10

NUTRITION

JULIE BOYER, RD

Adequate nutritional support is an integral part of a cancer patient's treatment. Nutritional problems in the cancer patient result from two causes: the systemic and localized effects of the disease itself and the specific treatment modalities. Malnutrition can complicate the clinical course and outcome of treatment; therefore, early intervention of nutritional support is important to impede the development of cancer cachexia. Studies have shown that adequate nutritional support may improve immunocompetence in patients treated with radiation or chemotherapy and that good nutritional status may increase response rates to therapy and also help promote better tolerance to the therapy.

Assessment

The major focus of this section is on nutritional assessment, that is, determining a patient's nutritional status and needs, and on enteral and parenteral methods of nutritional support. Malnutrition is an unacceptable consequence of cancer. It can be prevented by planning the therapeutic regimen so that nutritional support is adequate for the patient's changing nutritional needs in different phases of care.

Management of patients' nutritional care requires ongoing assessment of their nutritional status and begins with the preliminary nutritional screening. This screening is conducted to determine if there is need to evaluate more specific aspects of a patient's current nutritional status. A nutritional care plan is then formulated.

The preliminary nutritional screening first determines whether a patient is at risk of developing malnutrition. The information required includes results of the SMA 12 or SMAC and a CBC with a differential and what can be learned from the patient interview. Indications of risk for malnutrition secondary to cancer are serum albumin less than 3.5 gm/dl and total lymphocyte count less than 1500 prior to initiation of therapy; unplanned weight loss greater than 10 percent of normal body weight in the past six months; and eating problems including one or more of the following:

- anorexia;
- chewing or swallowing difficulties;
- change in taste or smell sensations;
- nausea, vomiting; and
- diarrhea, constipation.

The presence of two or more risk factors in the preliminary screening indicates that the patient is at risk for developing or may have a form of malnutrition. There are two choices of action:

1. Re-evaluate the patient in one week or at the next scheduled appointment to determine if there is any weight loss.
2. Immediately refer the patient for a diagnostic assessment basic to establishing a nutritional plan of care. Goals are to prevent further deterioration and assist the patient with dietary planning.

The patient's nutritional status and needs are determined in a diagnostic nutritional assessment. The nutritional assessment includes:

- a nutritional history,
- observation of physical signs of malnutrition,
- anthropometric measurements, and
- biochemical information.

Many parameters are used because no single one can measure nutritional status.

Information obtained in the nutritional history is used to evaluate the patient's past and present status. The following are typical questions asked in the interview.

1. What were your dietary patterns prior to illness?
2. What are your current dietary problems?
3. What were your dietary patterns during any past treatments?
4. What was your weight prior to illness? What is your present weight?
5. Have you noticed any changes in your eating habits? Anorexia? Taste or food preference changes?
6. Do you have difficulty chewing or swallowing?
7. Have you experienced nausea, vomiting, or diarrhea recently? What seems to cause these symptoms?

This subjective information is an important component of the preliminary nutritional screening and in the diagnostic assessment. It indicates the patient's current nutritional status and provides information used to develop a nutritional care plan, particularly for choosing a method of feeding.

CLINICAL EXAMINATION OF PHYSICAL SIGNS
Physical signs provide valuable information in determining nonspecific nutritional deficits that may be associated with vitamin, mineral, and protein-caloric deficiencies. Some physical signs possibly associated with malnutrition are listed in Table 10-1.

ANTHROPOMETRIC MEASUREMENTS
Next in the diagnostic assessment are the anthropometric measurements, which examine height and weight, protein and fat stores, and biochemical data from an examination of the visceral protein compartments. The patients' protein status directly affects their ability to respond to stress. Protein status is measured by the somatic proteins or muscle stores and the visceral proteins, which are all other proteins, such as serum proteins, enzymes, and hormones.

The somatic proteins directly affect work tolerance, deep breathing, coughing, and other respiratory and muscle coordinating functions. This compartment is assessed by height, weight, arm muscle circumference, and creatinine height index.

SOMATIC PROTEIN COMPARTMENT
The weight ideally is determined by direct measurement and compared to normal weight—the patient's weight prior to illness. Weight loss is a significant indicator of survival in cancer patients. Survival rates for patients who lost weight before chemotherapy are only about one-half that of patients who did not lose weight.

TABLE 10-1 PHYSICAL SIGNS ASSOCIATED WITH MALNUTRITION

Hair	Dry, dull, thin, straight, and easily plucked. Shows lighter or darker spots.
Face	Swollen. Dark cheeks and dark areas under eyes. Skin on nose and mouth lumpy and flaky. Enlarged parotid glands.
Eyes	Dull. Membranes dry and either too pale or too red. Triangular, shiny gray spots on conjunctivas, eyelid corners red and fissured. Bloodshot ring around cornea.
Lips	Red and swollen, especially at corners of mouth.
Tongue	Swollen. Appears raw, purple, with swollen sores or abnormal papillae.
Teeth	Missing or emerging abnormally. Cavities or dark spots showing. Gums spongy and bleed easily.
Neck	Thyroid glands swollen.
Skin	Dry, flaky, swollen, dark with lighter or darker spots, some resembling bruises. Skin appears tight and drawn.
Nails	Spoon-shaped, brittle and ridged.
Physique	Muscles wasted, legs knock-kneed or bowed, bumps on ribs, joints swollen.
Internal changes	Heart rate above 100, enlarged heart, abnormal rhythm, high blood pressure. Enlarged liver and spleen. Musculoskeletal hemorrhages.
Nervous system	Patient is irritable and confused, experiences burning and tingling of hands and feet, loss of sense of position and decreased ankle and knee reflexes.

Weight loss significant for nutritional-assessment purposes is defined as short-term—6 to 12 months—and involuntary. Weight loss greater than 10 percent is a significant weight loss; 20–30 percent is life-threatening. You can calculate the percentage of weight loss by dividing the difference between the patient's pre-illness weight and current weight by the pre-illness weight and multiplying by 100.

Anthropometric measurements are used to determine both fat stores and muscle mass. Triceps skinfold measurements (TSF) of the non-dominant arm are taken with a caliper. This measurement is a good indicator of body fat (calorie reserves), since approximately 50 percent of the adipose tissue is located in the subcutaneous area. The arm muscle circumference (AMC) is an indication of lean body mass or muscle tissue and is determined indirectly by figures derived from the midarm circumference and triceps skinfold. These values are compared to standards, and the percent deficits are determined. The TSF and AMC should be repeated weekly, although significant changes do not occur before three to four weeks. Determining muscle stores from these routes of measurement yield good baseline figures to use for future comparison, but are not totally accurate for evaluating actual muscle stores.

It may be difficult to obtain accurate arm measurement in breast cancer patients who have associated lymphedema in the nondominant arm. In these patients, it is acceptable to measure the other arm, unless both arms are edematous.

Creatinine, a normal metabolic byproduct of muscle, is excreted in the urine at a constant rate for a given quantity of muscle mass, regardless of a patient's metabolic state. The creatinine height index thus reflects the amount of lean body mass. A 24-hour urine creatinine is collected, and the quantity of urine creatinine excreted is compared to the expected 24-hour urinary creatinine excretion of a normal male or female of the same height. Patients with decreases in the lean body mass have decreases in urinary creatinine. However, results of the 24-hour urine creatinine test can be altered by abnormal renal function and insufficient fluid intake, as well as inaccurate urine collection.

Because the two components necessary to build skeletal muscle are the substrate protein and neuromuscular stimuli, the patient's CHI is improved by increasing physical activity.

VISCERAL PROTEIN COMPARTMENT
The visceral protein compartments are all proteins, excluding muscle mass. Deficits adversely affect patients' ability to respond to stress and are evidenced in slow wound healing and weakened immune response.

The visceral protein compartment is measured by serum albumin, serum transferrin, and total lymphocyte count. Serum albumin and transferrin are manufactured by the liver and both are sensitive to protein deprivation and hepatic function. Normal serum albumin levels range above 3.5 gm/dl. Lower values indicate deficits in the visceral protein compartment.

The serum half-life of albumin is 20 days and, therefore, serum albumin levels can reflect the quality and quantity of protein intake. Serum albumin, however, can also be affected for other reasons, including increased losses from renal or gastrointestinal disease, decreased synthesis due to liver disease, and hemodilution or concentration of the blood.

Hypoalbuminemia occurs frequently in cancer patients due to suppressed albumin synthesis, which may be a manifestation of the systemic effects of cancer.

Serum transferrin, the protein that transports iron, has a half-life of eight to 10 days and, therefore, is more sensitive to immediate changes in nutrition. Transferrin is best measured directly by obtaining a serum transferrin level, or indirectly by obtaining total iron binding capacity and using the formula $0.8 \times TIBC - 43 =$ serum transferrin. An increasing serum transferrin level reflects an improving nutritional status. As with any other parameter, serum transferrin can be affected by iron deficiency, anemia, blood loss, infection, and chronic disease.

Total lymphocyte count (TLC) may be useful in predicting a patient's ability to respond to infection. Lymphocytes, a type of leukocyte, function in the host's cellular immunity. A TLC is calculated from information provided by a CBC with differential, a factor determined by multiplying the white blood cell count by the percent lymphocyte, as illustrated in the formula: percent lymphocyte $\times$ WBC/100 = TLC. Levels below 1500 mm indicate decreased ability to respond appropriately to infection.

TLC can be affected by stress, steroids, chemotherapy, and radiation therapy. Therefore the validity of the measurement is decreased while a patient is receiving these treatments.

Another component of a nutritional assessment is delayed hypersensitivity skin tests or cell-mediated immunity. Cell-mediated immunity is an essential part of a patient's defense against infection. Immunoincompetence or anergy is associated with malnutrition and with increased morbidity and mortality.

Immunocompetence is determined by the host's response to at least one of four skin tests. Common antigens used are SK/SD (streptokinase/streptodormase), mumps, *Candida*, PPD, and trycophytan. Antigens are injected intradermally, usually on the forearm, and the area is checked at 24- and 48-hour intervals. If there is no response to at least one skin antigen within 24–48 hours, the patient is considered to be immunoincompetent or anergic. An anergic response can also be exhibited with the use of chemotherapeutic agents, immunosuppressants, and steroids.

Immunocompetence can be lost in seven days and restored approximately in two weeks with adequate nutrition.

NITROGEN BALANCE

The type of nutritional support required by a patient is determined in part by evaluation of nitrogen balance. A nitrogen balance study provides information for the initial plan of nutritional therapy and for subsequent evaluation of the adequacy of therapy.

The patient's nitrogen balance is studied to evaluate the adequacy of protein intake. About 16 percent of protein is nitrogen, and nitrogen excretion can be measured in urea nitrogen in the urine. About 95 percent of nitrogen is excreted in the urine, of which 80 to 90 percent is urea. The remaining 5 percent of nitrogen is excreted through the skin or stool.

Nitrogen balance is studied by comparing nitrogen intake and output. If protein is being catabolized for energy, the patient has a negative nitrogen balance, which indicates that nutritional support is insufficient. A positive nitrogen balance indicates that protein intake is being conserved and utilized for repair of protein deficits.

Because protein consists of 16 percent nitrogen, the intake of nitrogen can be determined by measuring protein intake, including both enteral and parenteral sources. Nitrogen output is determined from measurement of urea nitrogen in a 24-hour urine collection and by estimating the loss of nitrogen through skin and stool. Nitrogen balance is computed by using this formula: Nitrogen balance = (protein intake ÷ 6.25) − urine urea nitrogen + 4. Protein intake is calculated from a protein/calorie count taken during the 24-hour urine collection. The factor "4" used in this formula accounts for the estimated quantity of nitrogen loss through skin and stool. This loss is difficult to quantify and is higher if the patient has diarrhea, large wounds, fistulas, or burns.

Nitrogen equilibrium refers to nitrogen intake equal to nitrogen output resulting in a 0 to +2 nitrogen balance factor. Negative factors indicate that protein intake is insufficient for the patient's needs. A positive nitrogen balance results in values of +4 to +6 and indicates that protein is being conserved by the body. Because the effect of tumor growth on nitrogen balance is not well understood, a nitrogen balance study in a person with cancer may be less significant than in other persons. Consequently, a nitrogen balance study in a patient with cancer is used only as a guide to nutritional therapy and is considered along with other indicators of nutritional status.

NUTRITIONAL AND METABOLIC PROFILE
Once collected, the data from all tests are organized into a nutritional/metabolic profile. This profile aids in the diagnosis of the type and degree of malnutrition, which include kwashiorkor-like protein and marasmus forms of malnutrition.

Kwashiorkor-like protein malnutrition is caused by a diet consisting mainly of carbohydrate. Generally, this type of malnutrition has a rapid onset and is often seen in hospitalized patients who receive IV dextrose as their only calorie source. The typical profile in this form of malnutrition is preservation of somatic protein, normal anthropometric measurements, and depleted visceral proteins, possibly causing edema, which can mask weight changes. Immunoincompetence may also be

TABLE 10-2 COMPARISON OF TWO TYPES OF MALNUTRITION

Clinical features	Kwashiorkor	Marasmus
Visceral	Decreased	No change
Somatic	No change	Decreased
Onset	Rapid	Gradual
Type of malnutrition	Protein	Protein/calorie
Assessment	Frequently overlooked	Visually depleted

present. Because somatic protein is preserved, the patient's nutritional problem can be overlooked.

Marasmus is protein-calorie malnutrition. A decrease in adequate protein and calorie intake results in a gradual muscle wasting; in this event, a patient's muscle is obviously depleted. Clinical features include decreased somatic proteins, preservation of the visceral proteins, and possible immunoincompetence.

The most advanced stage of malnutrition and the most serious is the combination of marasmus and kwashiorkor, which is the depletion of both the somatic and visceral proteins. Additionally, immunoincompetence exists, and there is deterioration of the multiple organ systems, which make the care of this patient more complex. Table 10-2 provides a comparison of kwashiorkor and marasmus.

NUTRITIONAL PLAN OF CARE

Following assessment of the patient's nutritional status, the nutritional plan of care is established. Depending on the patient's status, nutritional support goals are either maintenance or repair of the protein compartments. The three major categories of nutritional status are shown in Table 10-3. As indicated in this table, the types of nutritional plans vary according to the category of malnutrition.

1. If patients have no nutritional deficits, but their condition places them at a nutritional risk, the goal is to maintain nutritional status. The nutritional management depends on the appetite or gastrointestinal function or both.
2. If the somatic and/or visceral proteins are depleted, the goal is to replenish, with a +4 to +6 nitrogen balance. Use of enteral or parenteral hyperalimentation is appropriate to ensure ingestion of needed protein and calories.
3. A hypermetabolic patient with or without nutritional deficits requires a neutral to greater than +4 nitrogen balance. Enteral or parenteral hyperalimentation is effective.

TABLE 10-3 KINDS OF NUTRITIONAL STATUS AND MANAGEMENT

Nutritional status	Examples	Goal	Nutritional management
No nutritional deficits, but clinical condition places person at nutritional risk	Chemotherapy Radiation Five days NPO Stroke	Maintain neutral N balance	Depends on appetite and GI function, diet supplementation, enteral or parenteral feedings or combination
Somatic and/or visceral protein deficits	Anorexia nervosa Cachexia	+ 4 to + 6 N balance	Enteral or parenteral hyperalimentation: 40–45 kcal/kg IBW; 1.5–2 gm protein/kg IBW
Hypermetabolic with or without nutritional deficits	Trauma, burns, surgery, infection	Neutral to + 4 N balance, depending on need for tissue repair	Enteral or parenteral hyperalimentation: up to 55 kcal/kg IBW; 2 + gm protein/kg IBW

Nutritional assessment continues as an integral part of the patient's care after completion of the initial diagnostic assessment or implementation of nutrition support. Repeated assessments are important to determine whether the objectives of the nutritional support are being met, and patients are monitored during all phases of care.

The American Society for Parenteral and Enteral Nutrition has formulated a specific protocol for patient monitoring. The guidelines for follow-up assessements are:

- daily—weights;
- weekly—total lymphocyte count, serum albumin, and serum transferrin;
- twice weekly—nitrogen balance; and
- biweekly—anthropometric measurements and skin testing.

Weight gain needs to be monitored to ensure that it is not due to fluid. A weight gain of 0.5 lb per day with parenteral nutrition and 0.7 lb per day with enteral nutrition is expected if adequate protein and calories are being provided.

Diagnostic assessments are not always possible; therefore, the preliminary nutritional screening procedure can be a useful tool to determine whether a patient is at risk for developing nutritional problems, and to interrupt this process early by implementing an appropriate nutritional care plan through multidisciplinary planning of care by the physician, dietitian, and nurse.

Nutritional support

In considering the method to be used for nutritional support, the general rule is: "If the gut works, use it." The three routes of nutritional support to be considered are:

- oral feedings with or without use of nutritional supplements;
- enteral (tube) feedings; and
- parenteral nutrition and use of intravenous amino acids, dextrose, and/or lipids.

Optimally, a patient's nutritional requirements should be met through oral intake. But anorexia and other side effects caused by the cancer or therapies frequently make it difficult for a patient to obtain sufficient protein and calories, causing the body to catabolize its own stores for energy. The effect is a caloric deficit, leading to weight loss. The patient should be taught early in the treatment phase about the importance of adequate nutrition and the nutritional goals during therapy. Patients who develop nutritional problems require assistance in learning about and using alternate solutions to maintaining a good nutritional status. This assistance is directed to helping the patient manage his or her individual problems.

It often happens that a patient asks, "Why do I have to eat, especially when I don't feel like it?" Patients who become aware of the benefits of optimal nutrition better accept the importance of nutrition as an integral part of therapy. Patients should actively participate in their nutritional care planning, which should begin early in the initial course of treatment. The benefits of optimal nutrition during treatment, ensuring adequate protein and calories are to:

- prevent or reverse weight loss;
- maintain ability to fight infection;
- allow better tolerance and possibly a more positive response to treatment;
- aid in repair of damaged tissues; and
- create an improved sense of well-being and strength.

Patients tend to treat nutrition as an integral part of their therapy when they know about and understand nutritional goals. These goals are similar to goals all healthy people should use to maintain good

TABLE 10-4 BASIC FOUR FOOD GROUPS

Group	Foods included	Daily amount required
Dairy	Milk, all cheeses, ice cream, yogurt	Adults require two cups per day or the equivalent of other milk products.
Meat (protein)	Meat (lamb, pork, beef), fresh poultry, eggs, or alternatives—dry peas, beans, peanut butter	Two 3-oz. servings per day.
Vegetables and fruit	All fruits including citrus fruit or juice; dark green or yellow vegetables	Four or more servings per day; include one citrus daily.
Bread and cereal	All breads and cereals that are whole grain enriched or restored; rice, noodles,	Four or more servings per day.

nutrition during the life cycle. However, the requirements for protein and calories are increased when the body is undergoing additional stress of either illness or treatment. The three basic nutritional goals for all to achieve are:

- eat a balanced diet;
- eat a high protein/high calorie diet; and
- maintain normal weight.

Each of these goals has implications for selection of foods.

A WELL-BALANCED DIET.
Choosing food from the basic four food groups to provide a diet with a variety of foods is the first step in ensuring a well-balanced nutrient intake (Table 10-4).

A HIGH-PROTEIN/HIGH-CALORIE DIET
The combination of protein and calories is important; they are both needed for body repair. Caloric needs increase approximately 20 percent. Adequate calories must be provided from carbohydrates and fats to allow for the functional use of the protein.

A patient's protein requirements may increase from 1.5 to 2.0 times normal needs as a result of the stress of illness. Protein is the functional component of the diet, used for repair or replacement of damaged cells. Therefore, a high-protein diet must be accompanied by the ingestion of sufficient nonprotein calories. To achieve this goal, the cancer patient who has lost his or her appetite must select each food to provide the maximum amount of nutrients in the smallest possible volume. Listed below are some suggestions to boost protein and caloric intake, but with minimal volume.

Calorie boosters

1. Fats are a good source of calories without adding volume:

   - Butter—use on vegetables, starches, hot cereals.
   - Mayonnaise—use in salads, sandwiches.
   - Sour cream and cream cheese—use in sauces, on potatoes and vegetables
   - Peanut butter—spread on fruit, such as apples and bananas, or use in sandwiches or on crackers; also a protein source.
   - Gravies

2. Carbohydrates are good in-between-meal snacks.

   - Add jelly or honey to toast, cottage cheese, hot tea, or hot cereal.
   - Popsicles, sherbet.
   - Drink juices instead of water.

Protein boosters

Many cancer patients develop an aversion to red meats; therefore, other foods are selected to ensure sufficient protein intake.

1. Milk: Add skim milk powder to whole milk. Use double-strength milk made by adding one-fourth cup of nonfat dry milk powder to one cup milk when milk is used for drinking, on cereal, in sauces, gravies, puddings, cream soups.
2. Meat, fish, poultry: Those patients who have an aversion to red meats can usually tolerate chicken and fish. Add small pieces to soups, casseroles, or use with sauces and gravies.
3. Cheese is a good source of protein that is usually well-accepted. Add grated cheese to cream sauces, casseroles, or vegetables. Use cottage cheese with fruit. Serve on crackers with juice for an excellent snack.
4. Eggs are another excellent and versatile source of protein. Blend finely chopped eggs into gravies and salad. Use in milkshakes or eggnogs.
5. Legumes: Soybean products, garbanzos, lentils—good source of protein if served with milk or grains.

TABLE 10-5 DETERMINING CALORIC NEEDS

Nutritional needs	To maintain weight	To gain weight
Calories	Actual kg body weight × 30–35	Actual kg body weight × 40–45
Protein	Actual kg body weight × 1	Actual kg body weight × 1.5–2

MAINTAIN WEIGHT

Often the goal of maintaining weight is difficult to achieve, especially when a patient is on a combination of therapies, for each therapy may affect the body differently. Maintenance of weight usually indicates that adequate calories and protein are being consumed. Helpful suggestions to maintain or gain weight are:

- small frequent feedings; for example, every two hours for a total of six meals or snacking;
- use protein/calorie booster ideas;
- don't fill up on low-calorie foods—drink juices instead of water, coffee, or tea;
- use nutritional supplements or milkshakes with or between meals;
- make the best of the "good days"; and
- keep a diet diary of food intake to determine calorie/protein intake.

Table 10-5 provides formulas to determine the patient's nutritional needs for calories and protein to either maintain or gain weight.

Frequently, the desire or ability to eat is decreased by the side effects of the cancer or the treatment modalities. These side effects include anorexia, taste changes, nausea and vomiting, dryness of mouth, stomatitis and esophagitis, diarrhea and constipation. Patients should be helped to find successful ways of treating these symptoms so that nutritional goals can be achieved. Table 10-6 includes some common complaints associated with cancer treatment side effects and some possible solutions that may be useful.

NUTRITIONAL SUPPLEMENTS

When patients are unable to consume adequate calories in the normal diet, they may be given liquid nutritional supplement. The nutritional supplement may be chosen from either commercially available formulas or can be prepared in the home or hospital setting to meet an individual patient's specific needs. The quantity of supplement needed is an important factor in selection, as is the patient's preference. Individualization in selection of supplements that both satisfies and meets the patient's nutritional needs improves the patient's willingness to consistently take the required quantity.

In individualizing nutritional therapy, calorie and protein needs are determined and compared to the patient's actual consumption of foods as observed and calculated by conducting a calorie/protein count or by diet history. Caloric deficit can be overcome by incorporating a specified quantity of one or more nutritional supplements into the diet. The effectiveness of oral supplementation depends on an individual's acceptance and motivation. Patients can sample the various supplements to determine their preferences. Serving the beverages well-chilled and when the patient wants them are helpful in achieving therapy goals. To avoid intolerance, a patient should be instructed to sip the beverages; to avoid taste fatigue and to maintain acceptability, the patient may interchange types of supplements that meet designated requirements.

Continued reinforcement about the vital role of nutrition in the treatment of cancer can be helpful in achieving the patient's cooperation when using the oral route as the method of choice.

ENTERAL NUTRITION

For those patients whose gastrointestinal tracts are functional, but who are unable to meet their nutritional requirements through oral intake, the use of a feeding tube is indicated. These are patients who find it difficult or are unable to swallow because of cancer of mouth, pharnyx, or esophagus, or who are unable to maintain adequate intake due to anorexia, or because of increased nutritional requirements during hypermetabolic states. Under these circumstances, a small soft feeding tube can be introduced into several sites along the alimentary tract. The tube can be passed through the nasal passages into the stomach, which acts as a reservoir controlling the release of formula into the intestines, or through the nasal passages into the duodenum or jejunum, bypassing the gastric esophageal and pyloric sphincters to avoid gastric reflex. Feeding tubes can also be placed directly into the stomach through a gastrostomy or into the jejunum through a jejunostomy. The gastrostomy tube is commonly used in patients who require long-term tube feedings. When feedings are placed directly into the stomach, the complete digestive and absorptive processes still occur.

Jejunostomy tubes are usually placed in those patients with problems that preclude use of direct feeding to the stomach. These include gastric carcinoma, chronic nausea and vomiting, and surgical intervention.

The jejunum cannot function as a reservoir and thus accepts less volume than does the stomach, so the volume rate and osmolality of the formula must be appropriately adjusted. Continuous drip feeding

Continued on page 214.

TABLE 10-6 COMMON COMPLAINTS AFFECTING NUTRITION

Anorexia

Cause: Disease process, treatment modalities, pain, and depression may decrease appetite.

Solutions:
- Six to eight small meals; high-calorie, high-protein snacks.
- Serve foods with attractive color and good texture; use smaller plates.
- Make eating a pleasurable experience with bright surroundings and companionship. Play soft music; have flowers on the table.

Taste changes

Cause: Some treatment modalities and the process of disease cause complaints of bitter or metallic tastes and lack of ability to taste. Decreased enjoyment of red meats is common.

Solutions:
- Experiment with various spices and flavoring to heighten flavors. Marinate foods in soy sauce, wine, or fruit juices. Tart foods—lemon or orange juice, vinegar—help to enhance flavors. Use strong seasonings—basil, oregano, curry, mint, rosemary.
- Substitute red meats for chicken or fish, dairy products, and eggs.
- Serve foods with attractive color and good texture.

Nausea and vomiting

Cause: Anticancer therapies can affect the part of the brain that stimulates nausea and vomiting. Emotional stress increases these symptoms.

Solutions:
- Antinausea medication administered one-half to one hour prior to meals.
- Meals should be eaten slowly.
- Avoid fluids with meals, drink fluids one hour before or after meals.
- Don't lie flat for at least two hours after eating.
- Drink cool or chilled beverages, such as carbonated beverages and fruit juice, slowly.
- Choose low-fat foods; avoid greasy or fried foods.
- Eat dry crackers or toast in the morning to help calm nausea.
- Avoid eating at times when nausea frequently occurs.
- Smell of foods frequently causes nausea. Choose cold foods or foods at room temperature; have someone else cook.

Dryness of mouth

Cause: Decreased salivation occurs during or after radiation of the head and neck area, causing difficulty in swallowing.

Solutions:
- Sip liquids with meals.
- Use gravies, cream, cheese sauces, butter on meats and vegetables, stews and casseroles.
- Use artificial saliva prescribed by physician.
- Stimulate salivation with hard lemon candy or hot tea with lemon.

Stomatitis and esophagitis

Cause: Mouth and throat areas are very sensitive to chemotherapy and radiation therapy, causing inflammation.

Solutions:
- Avoid acid, salty, spicy, or rough foods.
- Eat a soft, bland diet, using milkshakes, eggs, custards, puddings, cottage cheese, yogurt, nutritional supplements.
- Cold foods can be soothing.
- Avoid alcoholic beverages.

Diarrhea

Cause: Intestinal mucosa is frequently irritated by surgery, radiation to the abdominal area, or use of chemotherapeutic agents. Since the turnover rate of gastrointestinal cells is rapid, therapies can contribute to diarrhea.

Solutions:
- Eat a diet low in fiber. Choose only cooked fruits and vegetables and refined grains; avoid those with tough skin and seeds, whole grains.
- Avoid gas-producing foods, such as broccoli, cauliflower, corn, carbonated beverages. Do not chew gum.
- Avoid fatty or greasy foods.
- Drink low-acid juices: apricot, peach, pear nectars.
- Avoid milk products; they may not be tolerated at this time.
- Replace fluids and electrolyte losses. Apricot and peach nectar are high in potassium.

Constipation

Cause: Largely caused by narcotic analgesics and chemotherapeutic agents. Also influenced by low-fiber diet or liquids and decreased activity.

Solutions:
- Choose foods high in fiber: raw fruits and vegetables, whole grains, nuts, dried fruits.
- Increase fluid intake to at least eight glasses per day.
- Drink prune juice or hot lemon water in the morning or at night. Hot liquids often stimulate bowel function.
- Add one or two tablespoons bran to casseroles, hot cereals, milkshakes, baked goods. Bran is useful when a diet is limited to soft or liquid foods.

is used to prevent overloading the jejunum with a high volume of formula. An advantage of jejunostomy tube feeding is that it precludes the problem of gastric reflex.

As with selection of other dietary supplements, enteral nutrition is individualized according to the patient's condition and to goals of the nutrition therapy. The dietitian can help choose the appropriate diet. The following are points to consider in formula selection.

1. The patient's digestive and absorptive capabilities: Impaired digestion or absorption capacity may require partially digested formula—hydrolyzed proteins, free amino acids, simple sugars, low fat content.
2. Method and route of delivery.
3. Protein/caloric requirements: The majority of the commercial formulas are 1 cal/cc but can contain up to 2 cal/cc.
4. Electrolyte, vitamin, mineral, and trace element requirements:
   • Occasionally, electrolyte restrictions are necessary.
   • Vitamins, minerals, and trace elements are usually sufficient in a specified quantity of feeding solution but they can be added if normal requirements are not met or are greater.
5. Fluid requirements: Additional water may be required or the fluid can be decreased by increasing the concentration of the formula.
6. Other medical conditions that influence formula selection are:
   • lactose intolerance, allergies; and
   • diabetes and cardiac, renal, and liver disease.

In choosing a formula to fit the individual needs, it is necessary to know about the numerous products available. The feedings can be divided into several categories to be considered when choosing a formula (Table 10-7).

PARENTERAL NUTRITION

Parenteral nutrition is a nutritional support system to provide adequate nutrients intravenously. This type of nutrition therapy is used to maintain or restore body weight when feeding by way of the enteral route is contraindicated or inadequate. There are two general categories of parenteral nutrition—peripheral vein nutrition and parenteral hyperalimentation through a central vein. Both systems can be formulated with levels of nutrients specific to a patient's needs.

Peripheral vein nutrition is useful, provided the patient has good peripheral veins. Peripheral vein nutrition can be used only on a temporary basis to maintain nutrition; it cannot be used to meet increased requirements during states requiring nutritional repair or during hypermetabolic states.

TABLE 10-7 ENTERAL FORMULAS

Meal replacements—nutritionally complete formulas

A. Intact nutrient formulas require intact digestive and absorptive capacity.
- Calorie concentration: 1–2 cal/cc.
- Protein source varies: milk, soy, egg albumin.
- Fat content: Majority have moderate fat.
- Osmolality varies greatly: 300–690 mOsm/kg.
- Some palatable.
- Milk-based: Sustacal powder, Meritene.
- Lactose-free: 1 cal/cc—Ensure; Isocal; Osmolite; Precision LR, HN, and Isotonic.
  1.5 cal/cc—Ensure Plus, Sustacal HC.
  2 cal/cc—Magnacal, Isocal HCN.

B. Defined-formula diets: Partially digested nutrients requiring minimal digestion and used for patients with gastrointestinal dysfunction or in jejunostomy feedings.
- Calorie concentration: 1 cal/cc at full strength.
- Proteins: Hydrolyzed proteins, amino acids.
- Fats: Low-fat content, enough to provide essential fatty acids; some contain MCT oil.
- Limited palatability due to hydrolyzed protein and amino acids.
- Osmolality varies from moderate to high range: 450–800 mOsm/kg.
- Peptide/free amino acid formulas: Vital HN, Vipep, Criticare HN, Travasorb Peptide standard and HN.
- Crystalline amino acid formulas: Vivonex standard and HN.

Nutritionally incomplete

A. Defined-formula diets for specific metabolic conditions formulated for particular disease states.
- Renal insufficiency: Travasorb Renal, Amin Aid.
- Liver insufficiency: Hepatic Aid, Travasorb Hepatic.

B. Supplementary/modular feeding: Components of a feeding added to formula to increase a particular nutrient.
- Can be combined to create individualized feeding formula.
- Used to concentrate nutrients into small volume.
- Carbohydrates: Polycose, Cal-Power, HyCal, Moducal, Sumacal
- Fats: Lipomul, MCT oil
- Protein: Casec, Pro-Mix, Gevral Protein, Pro-Pac
- Combination: Citrotein, Controlyte

Indications for use include:

- a calorie and nitrogen source for supplementary use with an oral diet when a person will not take oral supplements or tube feeding;
- additional calories and nitrogen while a person is being introduced to enteral or parenteral hyperalimentation; and
- short-term maintenance calories and nitrogen for a person who is not hypermetabolic, but is taking nothing by mouth.

This system can be useful for the cancer patient to maintain nutritional status while receiving chemotherapy or radiation that causes severe nausea, vomiting, or diarrhea.

Central vein hyperalimentation is the most aggressive form of nutritional support. This system is designed to provide adequate nutrition by way of a central vein to those persons who cannot or should not be fed through the gastrointestinal tract. Indications for use include:

- a nonfunctional gastrointestinal tract, a need to keep the gastrointestinal tract at rest, or malabsorption problems;
- normal or increased nutritional requirements; and
- patients who cannot be managed adequately by peripheral vein nutrition or enteral hyperalimentation.

As with enteral feedings, nutritional adequacy is evaluated by frequent monitoring of a patient's nutritional status.

BIBLIOGRAPHY

Bistrian BR. Nutritional assessment and therapy of protein-calorie malnutrition in the hospital. J AM DIET ASSOC 71:393, 1977.

Blackburn GL, Bistrian BR, Maini BS, et al. Nutritional and metabolic assessment of the hospitalized patient. JPEN 1:11, 1977.

Blackburn GL. Nutritional assessment: An overview. CLIN CONSULT NUTR SUPPORT 1:1, 1981.

Chernoff R. Nutritional support: Formulas and delivery of enteral feedings. J AM DIET ASSOC 79:426, 1981.

Chicago Dietetic Association and South Suburban Dietetic Association. MANUAL OF CLINICAL DIETETICS, 2nd ed. Philadelphia: Saunders, 1981.

CONTEMPORARY PARENTERAL CARE OF THE CANCER PATIENT. North Chicago, Ill: Abbott Laboratories, 1980.

DeWys WD. Nutritional care of the cancer patient. JAMA 244:374, 1980.

Donaldson SS and Lenon RA. Impact of alterations of nutritional status: Chemotherapy and radiation therapy. CANCER 43:2036, 1979.

Heymsfield SB, Bethel RA, Ansley JD, et al. Enteral hyperalimentation: An alternative to central venous hyperalimentation. ANN INTERN MED 90:63, 1979.

Hooley RA. Clinical nutritional assessment: A perspective. J AM DIET ASSOC 77:682, 1980.

Kaminski, MV Jr. Enteral hyperalimentation. SURG GYNECOL OBSTET 143:12, 1976.

NURSING CARE OF THE CANCER PATIENT WITH NUTRITIONAL PROBLEMS. Columbus, Ohio: Ross Laboratories, 1981.

Shils ME. Enteral nutrition by tube. CANCER RES 37:2432, 1977.

———. Principles of nutritional therapy. CANCER 43:2093, 1979.

———. Nutritional problems induced by cancer. MED CLIN NORTH AM 63:1009, 1979.

Steffee WP. Cancer and protein malnutrition. COMP THER 3:9, 1977.

Theologides A. Cancer cachexia. CANCER 43:2004, 1979.

TUBE FEEDINGS: CLINICAL APPLICATIONS. Columbus, Ohio: Ross Laboratories, 1980.

Winborn AL, Banaszek NK, Freed BA, et al. A protocol for nutritional assessment in a community hospital. J AM DIET ASSOC 78:129, 1981.

Wollard JJ. NUTRITIONAL MANAGEMENT OF THE CANCER PATIENT. New York: Raven, 1979.

PATIENT EDUCATION MATERIALS

Akers S and Lenssen P. A GUIDE TO GOOD NUTRITION DURING AND AFTER CHEMOTHERAPY AND RADIATION, 2nd ed. Seattle: University of Washington, 1979. Available from Research Dietary Services, Department of Medical Oncology, Fred Hutchinson Cancer Research Center, 1124 Columbia St, Seattle, Wash 98104 ($3.50 per copy).

EATING HINTS: RECIPES AND TIPS FOR BETTER NUTRITION DURING TREATMENT. Washington DC: National Institutes of Health, 1980. Available from Superintendent of Documents, Government Printing Office, Washington, DC 20402 ($5.50 per copy).

Fishman JA, Anrod B, and Graham J. SOMETHING'S GOT TO TASTE GOOD: THE CANCER PATIENT'S COOKBOOK. Fairway, Kan: Andrews and McMeel, 1981.

Helsen JE. FOOD FOR THOSE WHO HESITATE—TIPS THAT THEY MAY TOLERATE. Available free from Cancer Information Center, Duke University Comprehensive Cancer Center, 200 Atlas St, Durham, NC 27705.

NUTRITION FOR PATIENTS RECEIVING CHEMOTHERAPY AND RADIATION TREATMENT. New York: American Cancer Society, 1974. Available free from local chapters of the American Cancer Society.

Rosenbaum EJ, Stitt C, Drasin H, et al. HEALTH THROUGH NUTRITION: A COMPREHENSIVE GUIDE FOR THE CANCER PATIENT. San Francisco: Alchemy, 1978.

11

PAIN MANAGEMENT

MARY E. MIELNICKI, RN, BSN

Pain control is one of the most complex aspects of the cancer patient's long-term care. The source of pain in cancer patients is the tumor, which can press on an organ such as the liver, directly involve the nerve plexus or the spinal cord, thereby interrupting sensory fibers, or, when bone is directly involved, cause periosteal irritation or pathologic fractures. Pain can also result from treatment. Both chemotherapy and radiation may cause fibroses or scarring of nerve fibers, causing direct pain.

The experience of pain varies among patients, depending partly on each one's physical, psychological, and environmental stimuli. Pain can be a protective mechanism; it occurs when body tissue is damaged and indicates a need to intervene to relieve pain. The sensation of pain varies according to the specific way stimuli cause pain in different body tissues. Pain varies also in quality, intensity, duration, severity, and in individual responses.

The pain threshold is individualized by factors such as inflammation that lower the threshold. Analgesics, distractors, or strong emotion increase the threshold.

The pain sensation is initiated by stimulation of pain receptors located throughout the body. Complex networks of pain pathways allow neural impulses to be transmitted through somatic and visceral nerves to the spinal cord, where they either terminate or are passed on to higher brain centers, some reaching the cortex. There is segmental innervation for peripheral pain pathways, allowing for reflex action at the level of the spinal cord. Nerve roots in the first to fourth segments of the spinal cord, for example, provide pathways for sensory fibers from the intrathoracic vertebrae. In addition, there are mixed, overlapping, and collateral pathways for transmission of pain impulses from the spinal cord to the brain which are not fully understood.

Factors that influence stimulation of nerve fibers are also complex. Pain mediators have been isolated that cause pain when released at the site of injury. Bradykinins, serotonin, histamine, and prostaglandins are examples of pain mediators. Certain chemicals, such as salicylates, may inhibit these mediators and thus they are analgesics. The perception of pain is similarly complex and is thought to result from networks of sensory fibers connecting the thalamus and the cortex.

Pain sensations also seem to persist as long as the stimuli continue, indicating that the awareness and perception of pain differ from other types of sensory stimuli for which there are negative adaptations; for example, the stimuli on the sense of smell do not exert a long-lasting effect.

Pain sensations, because they tend to be elicited by complex networks among higher brain centers, are not easily defined. Individual responses to pain probably are explained by the intricacies of the pain networks. Emotions like anxiety, anguish, depression, or nausea are elicited in the pain response. Physiologic responses such as vasoconstriction evidenced in pale, clammy skin, increased diastolic and systolic blood pressure, and increased respiratory rate are associated with pain responses. People vary in their personal response to pain; some are quiet, and others are verbal and tend to express their feelings readily. Fatigue or stress may influence the pain response.

Psychological Aspects of Pain

The sensation of pain is activated by complex neurophysical responses to stimuli, influenced by the patient's anxiety level, previous experiences with pain, and cultural, social, and environmental factors. Assessing pain response requires discussion with the patient to ascertain the relative importance of the many factors that may influence the sensation of pain and the resultant behavioral response. Knowledge of these factors is necessary to develop a comprehensive plan for the patient's pain control.

Basic to assessment of a patient's pain is that pain is whatever the patient perceives it to be. Some patients are able to verbalize their perceptions whereas others may be reluctant to disclose their feelings or lack the energy to do so. You can get information about the patient's perception of pain in an assessment interview, by talking with family members or others who can interpret his responses through their knowledge of his or her typical behavior, and by observing the patient's responses over time.

The following are questions you might ask the patient during the assessment interview:

- In what circumstances do you notice the pain?
- What seems to trigger the pain?
- How do you relieve the pain? What methods seem to work best for you?
- How does the pain interfere with your life?
- In your opinion, how do you emotionally react to pain? Does it cause you to be fearful or anxious?
- Do you anticipate the pain before it occurs?
- What type of relief do you expect from pain-control methods you are now using?

Your evaluation of the patient's answers to these and other questions is partly subjective, but you can also rely on your knowledge of the various ways people usually perceive and respond to pain. Because patients may use standard terms to describe pain, you need to ask probing questions to clarify what the patient actually means. With regard to relief from pain, for example, one patient's expectation may be total absence of pain. Some patients do not expect to be pain-free but may have adapted to a low-grade pain as a normal state. For some patients, pain control means decrease in fear or anxiety. Yet other patients may interpret pain control as meaning that they can perform activities, such as jogging or sewing. For many patients, pain interferes with the ability to concentrate; for them, pain control means being able to read a book or perform a task that requires concentration. Patients with long-term cancer experience the effects of decreased energy, and for these patients, pain control may mean being able to enjoy family dinners or visiting with good friends.

Personality influences how the patient expresses pain responses. Some patients are self-contained and don't readily express their feelings. In contrast, other patients talk freely of their experiences and will tell you everything they do when they experience pain. Other behaviors you may observe in a patient are helpful in evaluating his pain response. Some people favor or hold the painful body area. Others are quiet and may seem withdrawn when experiencing pain. Expressions of anger, becoming upset over trivial matters, or other indicators may be a better index of some patient's pain than verbal expression.

The purpose of assessment of the patient's perception of and response to pain is to understand the patient's behavior and to develop a plan for pain control that is individualized to the patient. When setting goals for pain control, you and the patient should consider options available. Inform the patient of available options, seek his or her opinions about each, and interpret possible effects of each option in practical terms. Even though there are typical responses to each method, this patient's response may differ. Let the patient know that methods of pain control can be altered according to need and options for pain control. Inform the patient of any expected side effects, limitations, or restrictions associated with each option. Certain analgesics, for example, result in decreased alertness, so the patient should not drive or operate machinery. The patient should know the limitations or restrictions before selecting an option for pain control.

Implementing a plan for pain control begins with the patient's agreement to it if feasible. Once it is begun, both you and the patient evaluate the effectiveness of the selected plan. Common understanding developed in planning aids evaluation of outcomes. Observe the patient's response to the pain-control method and also ask him or her to evaluate its effects. Your words and mannerisms may influence the patient's pain experience. If you ask, "How is your pain today?" or "Are you in pain?" the patient may register the word pain, which may lead to experiencing pain. Because patients may be suggestible, you should phrase questions in neutral terms. "How comfortable are you?" or "How do you feel today?" are expressions that the patient registers as comforting, thus leading to a sensation of comfort.

Nurses may become frustrated when a patient responds to pain by crying, or when a patient prefers to tolerate the pain quietly rather than seek help. You should assess your personal feelings about pain. Do you respect or are you frustrated by the patient who bears pain quietly. Your tolerance and acceptance of a patient's behavior in the face of pain can help you to be more objective in assessing the patient's response and, consequently, more effective in planning and implementing interventions.

Pain control is complicated. As patients move through phases of cancer, and as a patient's needs and expectations change, pain-control measures are evaluated and adjusted. Fundamental to this entire process is the quality of communication among members of the care team and the family unit, and, of course, between you and the patient.

Treatment of Pain

Depending on the source of pain stimuli and other variables, pain is treated in different ways. Analgesics, surgical intervention, radiation therapy, and psychologic approaches are used to help control pain. Each of these is described below.

ANALGESICS

Analgesics relieve or reduce pain without loss of consciousness. Analgesics can be classified as narcotic or nonnarcotic.

Nonnarcotics are medications that can be sold without a prescription; acetaminophen and aspirin are examples. Taken in large amounts, these nonnarcotic analgesics can cause severe side effects such as nausea, vomiting, and constipation. Nonnarcotics are used for relieving mild pain but are usually not sufficient in management of chronic pain. Although it is not totally clear how these analgesics work, current theories are that they inhibit pain mediators or interfere with the pain receptors, in the peripheral system.

Narcotics are drugs that require a prescription. If taken inappropriately, they can cause death. Their side effects vary; they can be addictive, and, when discontinued after extended use, withdrawal symptoms occur. Narcotics are thought to act mainly at the level of the higher brain centers. Narcotics and nonnarcotics frequently are combined in treatment. Examples of these combinations are Darvocet-N 50, which contains 50 mg propoxyphene napsylate and 325 mg acetaminophen, and Tylenol #3, which contains 30 mg codeine and 300 mg acetaminophen. There are many available medications containing a combination of narcotics and nonnarcotics. These combinations are effective because each analgesic has a different mechanism for relieving pain, and, by combining them, lower dosages of each are needed, reducing the side effects and risk of addiction while still maintaining pain control.

The following are questions to guide you in the selection of pain medication:

- Is the pain chronic or temporary?
- Is pain expected to decrease in the future, possibly by chemotherapy, radiation, or surgery?
- Is it probable the pain will increase in the future?
- Will pain control become a long-term management problem?
- What is the intensity of pain?
- How does the patient rate the pain, mild or very painful?

TABLE 11-1 FREQUENTLY USED ANALGESICS

Narcotic	Usual dose IM	PO	Duration	Peak	Onset	Side effects	Comments
	in mg		in hours	in min	in min		
Morphine	10	60	4–6	60	10–15	respiratory depression	Parenteral is route of choice
Meperidine	75	30	3–4	30–60	5–10	respiratory depression	Onset faster than morphine; good for acute pain.
Codeine	60	120	3–4	30–60	5–10	nausea, vomiting, constipation	Good choice for mild pain; often given with acetaminophen.
Levorphanol (Levo-Dromoran)	2	4	6–8	60–90	1	respiratory depression; less nausea than with other narcotics	Good for oral medication of severe pain.
Hydromorphone	2	6–8	3–4	60	5–10	hypotension	
Methadone	10	20	8–12	60–120	10	nausea, vomiting	Has been used successfully for tolerance of narcotics.

- What has the patient found effective for pain control in the past?
- What route of administration should be used? Will the patient be able to self-medicate? Can the patient tolerate oral medication?
- Do the patient's activities limit the use of analgesics that interfere with safety, such as driving a car or operating machinery?

These and other factors serve as guidelines for selection of pain medications most suitable for the patient's need to control pain while still maintaining maximum activity.

The most frequently used analgesics are presented in Table 11-1. The side effects listed in the table include only those that occur most frequently. In selecting the route of administration for analgesics, the patient's ability to take or tolerate oral medications and its effectiveness for pain control are assessed. Oral medication is the route of first choice, although most of the analgesic preparations for oral administration require larger doses than for parenteral administration. The advantage of oral administration is ease in self-medication.

SCHEDULING PAIN MEDICATIONS

Administration of pain medications may be either as needed (PRN) or routinely. Current evaluation studies indicate that routine schedules may provide for maintenance of a constant blood level of medication. Scheduled pain medication seems to be more effective for control of chronic pain.

A systematic method for determining the most appropriate schedule is using the PRN administration for 48 hours as a trial. Information obtained in this trial period is used to plan the patient's medication schedule. During the 48-hour trial period, the patient is instructed to keep a diary in which the following information is entered:

- the exact time the medication is taken for each dose;
- the exact amount taken;
- the pain level, as evaluated by the patient at the time the medication is taken, using a scale from mild to moderate to severe;
- the time the medication began to take effect;
- the pain-free period; and
- side effects, if any.

This information is used to establish a routine medication schedule to achieve a desired blood level.

In instructing the patient about self-medication, include information about side effects. Also inform the patient that certain circumstances, such as increased activity and stress, may temporarily change the time of effectiveness of a medication. The medication schedule and dosage are re-evaluated periodically as the patient's condition changes.

PARENTERAL ADMINISTRATION

Some patients may be unable to tolerate oral medications and require subcutaneous intramuscular injections. If the patient is unable to administer the injection, a family member or responsible person can be taught the correct procedure. The method used to determine schedules for oral medications may be used for establishing intramuscular administration schedules.

Narcotics are administered intravenously when the patient cannot take oral or intramuscular medications. In this event narcotics can be administered on a continuous 24-hour drip method. Morphine is most frequently given in this way. The following are likely candidates for continuous IV drip:

- patients in severe pain who do not experience relief from medication given at intervals;
- patients whose severe pain is estimated to be temporary, because future treatment—chemotherapy, radiation, or surgery, singly or in combination—is expected to decrease pain;
- patients whose illness is terminal and for whom the main goal is providing comfort.

The IV drip method is not appropriate for the patient who will return to the home environment at the same pain level.

There are no fixed rules for selection of either a pain medication or its route. The patient's experience is the best guide, because pain is a sensation influenced by complex interactions between physical and emotional factors. By definition, pain is what the patient feels.

RELAXATION

Relaxation techniques are used as part of pain-control plans. Often, a combination of relaxation techniques are incorporated in a comprehensive plan of analgesia, exercise, rest, and adequate nutrition, all of which influence the patient's feeling of well-being. Of the more commonly used relaxation techniques, self-hypnosis, imagery, meditation, and progressive relaxation exercises have proved effective for patients with cancer. In self-hypnosis, the patient learns to block outside stimuli and to focus on a positive image, thought, or scene. Self-hypnosis should be taught to patients by a reputable professional. Imagery is the procedure of focusing on an object while relaxing body muscles. Patients are able to learn imagery from an experienced guide.

Meditation is concentrating or focusing attention on a single thought or task. Progressive relaxation exercises may also be learned. The patient progressively relaxes and tenses muscles while concentrating on the changing tension. Depending on the patient's response pattern and preferences, a combination of techniques may be used. People vary in whether they respond best to music, touch, or visual stimuli, all of which may be used in relaxation techniques.

Before beginning a relaxation program, the patient's previous habits should be assessed. Find out how the patient has previously reduced stress or relaxed. The patient should be encouraged to continue using techniques known to be effective. Techniques new to the patient can be incorporated into a relaxation program, building on the patient's past experiences. After the patient has learned the techniques and has adapted them to his or her response patterns, help him to use them on a daily basis.

Surgery and Radiation

Surgical intervention to achieve pain control is used for patients for whom analgesics and psychologic interventions are not effective or who have intractable pain. The goal of surgical intervention is to either inhibit or interfere with the transmission of impulses to the central nervous system. Nerve blocks, cordotomy, or neurectomy are three commonly used procedures.

Nerve blocks. Injection of a local anesthetic close to a nerve blocks conduction of impulses. Depending on the medication used, nerve blocks can be reversible. In some patients, they are not successful. Because the source of the patient's pain and the perception of pain are complex, patients may require continued use of analgesics and relaxation techniques, even if the nerve block is successful. Complications of nerve blocks include infection, drug reaction, or, if an overdose of the drug is given, cardiac arrest.

Permanent pain relief. Cordotomy and neurectomy are among the procedures that may be used to achieve permanent pain relief. These procedures are used for patients whose pain is not relieved by narcotics and who probably will have long-term pain. In these procedures, the nerve is severed, as in cordotomy, or tissue around the nerve is destroyed to prevent passage of impulses. Complications of these procedures are paralysis, infection, and other side effects that are possible with any surgical procedure.

Radiation. Used as a palliative measure in pain control, radiation is especially effective for the pain caused by bony metastasis. Radiation decreases pain either by decreasing the size of the lesion or tumor causing pain or by destroying tissue cells around the nerve to inhibit nerve conduction. When used for pain control, radiation is given in low doses—usually 2500 to 3500 rads. The side effects of radiation are minimal and are usually localized or directly related to the area being radiated. Specific side effects of radiation are discussed in Chapter 4.

Ethical Issues

The management of pain, especially at the end stage of cancer, can present some difficult ethical issues for the nurse, who is most often the person controlling the management of pain for the patient. The nurse initially assesses the patient's pain control needs, decides how much and how often to give a pain medication that is ordered PRN, and is the person who most often helps decide to increase or change a narcotic.

The decisions of the person giving narcotics are often difficult and present an ethical dilemma. At the end stage of a disease process, comfort with regard to quality of life for the patient is the main goal. Intravenous narcotics such as meperidine or morphine are often used. The patient may not be alert or oriented at this point. The question of how much narcotic to give a patient is difficult to assess. Comfort versus the hastening of death becomes the issue.

There are no set rules or steps to follow when making these decisions. You must rely on your assessment skills. You need to assess the signs of pain for the patient. Does the patient's moaning mean pain, fear, or anxiety? Does the patient's constant movement mean pain or does it provide comfort?

The narcotic dosage should be increased slowly in order to decrease the effects of respiratory depression. Remember that your goal of treatment in the end-stage of advanced disease is to maintain comfort and not to prolong life.

But you should not feel pressured into administering a narcotic if you don't feel comfortable doing so. Share your concerns with other members of the medical team. If the consensus is to give a narcotic, support the team's decision in giving the medication.

Another role of the nurse during the end stage is to help the family members deal with the patient's pain. Often the movement or moaning of a patient can upset them. These signs mean pain to them. Teach the family members to realistically assess pain. Let them know when the last pain medication was given, how often a narcotic can be given, and that it can decrease respirations. Reassure family members that the medical team's goal is the patient's comfort and that they will achieve this goal as best they can.

BIBLIOGRAPHY

Bergersen BS. PHARMACOLOGY IN NURSING, 14th ed. St Louis: Mosby, 1979.

Burkhalter PK and Donley DL (eds). DYNAMICS OF ONCOLOGY NURSING. New York: McGraw-Hill, 1978.

Guyton AC. TEXTBOOK OF MEDICAL PHYSIOLOGY, 6th ed. Philadelphia: Saunders, 1981.

Luckmann J and Sorensen KC. MEDICAL-SURGICAL NURSING; A PSYCHOPHYSIOLOGIC APPROACH, 2nd ed. Philadelphia: Saunders, 1980.

McCaffery M. NURSING MANAGEMENT OF THE PATIENT WITH PAIN, 2nd ed. Philadelphia: Lippincott, 1979.

12

COMPLICATIONS: RECURRENCE OR METASTASIS AND INFECTION

MICHELLE A. McCLANAHAN, RN, BS

To the cancer patient and the health care team, metastasis evokes fear, anger, and dread of the future. Metastasis means that tumor cells have migrated from the primary site to a secondary site, another body part or organ. Evidence of metastasis may be found at the time of initial diagnosis or may be discovered several months or even years later. One of the principle goals of treatment for the oncology patient is to prevent further spread of the tumor cells.

Metastasis is confirmed through a variety of methods. In some patients, visible physical symptoms such as a bowel obstruction indicate metastasis. In others, metastasis is found through results of routine test procedures, such as a scan, X-ray or CEA-blood level.

There is continuous clinical research to discover how metastasis occurs and to identify factors that promote or inhibit this process. It has been found thus far that the spread of tumor cells from the primary site may occur through one or a combination of modes. They can be directly seeded into body cavities or implanted during surgery. The tumor cells may involve the lymphatic network and travel to a distal site. They may spread via the vascular system or infiltrate adjacent cavities. The exact mechanism of tumor spread via the lymphatics is unknown. A developing theory is that the tumor spreads via the interstitial planes toward the small lymphatic capillaries. Flow toward the lymphatics may be due to hydrostatic pressure, gravity, and actual tumor activity. Normally, the lymphatic valves prevent retrograde flow, thus permitting the nodes to act as filters for foreign materials. Lymphvenous anastomosis permits entry of tumor cells into the bloodstream. Not all tumors are able to spread, but those that do, spread at various rates. There is a wide range of predictability for cancer dissemination. Treatment of metastasis can be complicated when multiple sites are identified at the same time, thus making it difficult to isolate the primary from the secondary sites.

Tumor cells differ from normal cells in that they are motile, exhibit a decrease in surface "stickiness," and can migrate and easily lose connection with the parent growth. Also, tumor cells at the secondary site demonstrate characteristics different from those cells at the primary site. Metastatic cells are of a different size, vary in number, and their rate of proliferation may change. Through research, it has been found that differences in the surface properties of the metastatic cell may determine future spread. In addition to changes in their motility and adhesiveness, tumor cells produce lytic substances that may alter the adjacent tissues to facilitate infiltration. There still remains the question as to what causes the tumor cell to move.

Although the sites of metastasis vary according to the type and location of the primary tumor, the most frequent sites of metastasis are the bone, brain, lung, and liver. In metastasis to the bone, there is associated severe pain and gradual disability with the potential for pathological fractures. When the tumor spreads to the brain, the patient may experience headaches, seizures, mental changes, or other signs and symptoms. Metastasis to the liver is characterized by local congestion and development of ascites. With lung metastasis, the patient experiences difficulty in breathing and limitation of energy.

As mentioned previously, the extent of metastasis is evaluated at the time the initial diagnosis is made. However, the oncology patient requires follow-up diagnostic workup and testing to evaluate the effectiveness of therapy. Some require further treatment in an effort to control the disease and achieve either relief or management of the physical symptoms. In these situations, you will have repeated contact with patient and family. One of the most challenging and difficult aspects of oncology care is to give consistent psychological support. When metastasis occurs and the disease is progressive, the patient faces the fact that treatment is failing to control the disease.

Another major complication of metastasis develops when an effusion forms secondary to tumor involvement and infiltration. An effusion is formed when fluid accumulates in a body cavity or tissue. The two most commonly occurring sites for effusions are the pleural space or the peritoneal cavity. Treatment of effusions is directed toward drainage of the fluid and prevention of a recurrence. The physician may choose to instill cytotoxic agents to produce a chemical irritation and/or obliterate space to prevent recurrence. Examples of cytotoxic agents used include radioisotopes and alkylating or other chemotherapeutic agents. Treatment may require insertion of a chest tube for a pleural effusion or insertion of abdominal drains or a catheter for a peritoneal effusion.

Prevention of Infection

The development of an infection is one of the most frequently occurring life-threatening complications for oncology patients. The increased risk of infection results from disruption of the body's natural defenses, and this occurs for several reasons. The actual disease process alters the body functions, particularly the immune system. After major surgery, the body directs its energy toward healing the surgical wound. Chemotherapy and radiation therapy may induce bone-marrow depression and neutropenia. Also, with the development of technologial advances, such as the long-term placement of an intravenous catheter, new risks are always being introduced. In this section, the occurrence of events, their treatment, and nursing management of the patient are described.

DISRUPTION OF BODY DEFENSES

Bacterial and fungal infections develop when neutropenia exists. There is an inverse relationship between circulating granulocytes and frequency of infection. As circulating granulocytes decrease, the frequency of infection increases. When signs and symptoms of an infection occur, appropriate specimens are obtained for culture and the causative organism is identified. Antibiotic therapy may be started before culture results are obtained if the patient's condition warrants it.

Cell-mediated and humoral immunity are disrupted because of disease or therapy, making the patient vulnerable to bacterial or viral infections. Following a splenectomy, the body loses a natural protector; thus these patients are at risk for the incidence of infection.

The oncology patient is subject to environmental and iatrogenic risks of hospitalization, particularly at these critical times:

1. Postoperatively, there is danger of wound infection. Look for signs of it and make sure that the patient performs deep breathing exercises to avoid respiratory complications.

2. During the course of therapy, the patient may have various intravenous lines and drainage tubes. These invasive procedures place the patient at risk of infection.

Depending upon location and size, a tumor can cause an obstruction, thus predisposing the patient to infection.

TREATMENT AND NURSING CARE

In immunosuppressed patients, the usual signs of infection may be hidden. When their blood counts are low, these patients may require reverse isolation as a means of prevention and protection. Follow these guidelines for prevention of infection:

1. Do frequent physical assessments, which will enable you to detect signs of infection early.
2. Measure the patient's temperature frequently. The patient should be taught to continue this practice at home.
3. Instruct the patient about the necessity of good oral hygiene and the importance of dental check-ups with frequent inspection for mouth sores, gum integrity, and other risk factors.
4. Increase the patient's oral fluid intake.
5. Ensure sterile technique when handling all indwelling catheters, drainage tubes, and intravenous lines.
6. Teach the patient to avoid contact with persons who have colds or other contagious diseases, to avoid crowds, and immediately to report any symptoms to the physician.
7. Monitor CBCs on a regular basis. When a patient's white count, platelet count, and others fall to dangerously low levels, the patient is usually placed in reverse isolation. Reverse isolation requires that the patient be placed in a private room. All members of the health-care team and visitors are required to wear a gown, mask, and gloves before entering the room and caring for the patient. If the institution does not have facilities for isolation, a special cart with all of the necessary supplies should be located at the door of the patient's room. Also, reverse isolation signs should be placed on the door, the patient's chart, and Kardex. It is important to emphasize to the patient and family that reverse isolation is implemented for protection of the patient from others and not because the patient is "contaminated."
8. Reinforce the need for good nutrition, adequate rest, and vigilance in early detection of any minor sores or infections.

Members of the health care team should remain alert to the potential of infections as any new advance in oncology treatment is introduced.

BIBLIOGRAPHY

Bouchard R and Owens NF. NURSING CARE OF THE CANCER PATIENT, 4th ed. St Louis: Mosby, 1981.

Day SB, Stonsly P, Laird Myers WP, et al (eds). CANCER INVASION AND METASTASIS: BIOLOGIC MECHANISMS AND THERAPY. New York: Raven, 1977.

DeVita VT, Hellman S, and Rosenberg SA. CANCER—PRINCIPLES AND PRACTICE OF ONCOLOGY. Philadelphia: Lippincott, 1982.

Khandekar JD and Lawrence GA. FUNDAMENTALS IN CANCER MANAGEMENT. Niles, Ill: MEL 1982.

Lawrence W Jr and Terz JJ. CANCER MANAGEMENT. New York: Grune & Stratton, 1977.

METASTASIS AND DISSEMINATED CANCER. New York: American Cancer Society, 1979.

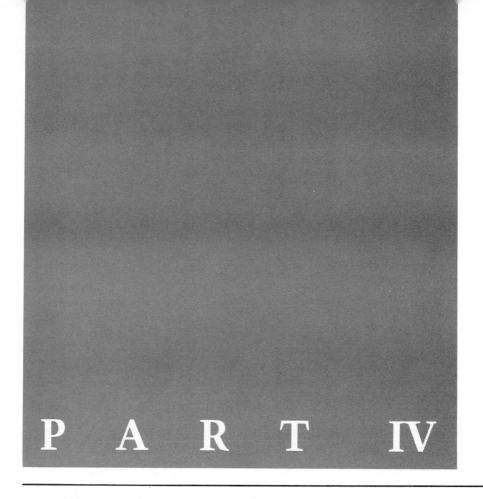

PART IV

SPECIAL
CONSIDERATIONS

13

ETHICAL ISSUES IN CANCER NURSING

SUZANNE DURBURG, RN, BSN, MEd

Health professionals are involved with ethics because some of their decisions in patient care matters are moral decisions. Health professionals also counsel patients, families, or persons responsible for patients in making choices about how they will participate in care activities. Ethics, the study and development of principles governing moral choice, provides guidance to effective decision-making and provides guidelines for resolving potential conflict surrounding this decision-making. Nurses and other health professionals are challenged to be effective participants in moral decision-making. Ethics provides a system of thought for confronting the overwhelming moral decisions that are part of patient care.

Medical Ethics

Medical ethics focuses on the morality of health-care decisions. Increasingly, interventions made possible by advancing medical technology complicate ethical decision making. Appropriate use of highly technologic interventions must be determined by patient-centered decisions. Both the health-care professional—the nurse or doctor—and the environment influence this decision making. The health professional's own self-interests and the environment where care is delivered can be obstacles to awareness of moral choices. Health-care providers must develop sensitivity to the moral choices they make and to the choices they counsel others to make.

To be true patient advocates, nurses must be open to examining their beliefs and value systems. This can help them better understand why they make the decisions they do and more fully develop the ability to identify moral conflicts and choices in themselves, their patients, and their patients' families.

THE PATIENT'S PERSPECTIVE

To become a patient is to become dependent on physicians and nurses in an environment they control. Patients are expected to abide by the rules of the hospital, to learn the codes of patient behavior that are often new to them but familiar to the physicians and nurses. Many patients adapt; they learn how to behave to obtain what they need. Some patients feel dehumanized or depersonalized in the hospital environment. Professional concern, warmth, reassurance, and comfort—all of which are part of nursing care—do not totally lessen the patient's dependence and its consequences. It is therefore imperative that nurses develop a broad perspective of medical ethics. In making moral choices, nurses must recognize the effects of "patienthood"; they must allow patients freedom to make their own choices within the context of the hospital environment and the patients' illness circumstances.

DEVELOPING ETHICAL POSITIONS

A person's values, norms, and beliefs of ethical principles are first unconsciously and then consciously formulated. Ethical principles are continuously examined in the light of new information about social and technologic issues. Nurses must be informed about the ethical component of care decisions because what is right or wrong, good or bad, often depends on the patient's circumstances.

It is not unusual for ethical principles to be interpreted as legal considerations. Unethical decisions by nurses and physicians make them subject to legal action by patients and families. To protect patients and professionals, decisions are posed in legalistic terms, stated as law to govern professional behaviors. But the nature of ethics requires that decisions be made in the patient's context. Ethical principles should be applied to the patient's situation.

Each profession may view the ethical decisions differently, however, because of the characteristics of the profession's mission. The result is debate about moral issues. The debate rages between physician and philosophers, consumers and the health-care establishment, and nurses and doctors. Each group brings its own perspective to the consideration of moral conflicts. For example, medical education concerns itself with cure of disease, and produces physicians who are biased toward continued aggressive intervention in the disease process in the patient. Nursing education concerns itself with care and assessing and meeting patients' needs. As a reflective physician said, "It is the physician who orders the chemotherapy for the patient, but the nurse holds the patient and the emesis basin when the side effects display themselves." These differences in perspective are important to recognize, for they guide ethical decisions. Medicine and nursing have professional codes of conduct that influence the behavior of each group in patient care.

In addition to each professional's perspective, the patient also has a personal perspective based on values, norms, and beliefs. In patient care activities the different perspectives interface, and professionals and patients come into conflict over ethical decisions and struggle with moral decisions. Professionals who approach these choices with a sense of their own vulnerable humanity serve their patients best.

PATIENT RIGHTS
For many reasons, mostly related to the consumer rights movement, there has been considerable attention paid to the rights of consumers of health care. The professions of medicine and nursing and the larger health-care industry have been challenged to relinquish paternalistic control over decisions regarding patient care and return decision making to patients and their families. Conflicts over who makes what decisions continually occur in hospitals and other health-care facilities.

The President's Commission for the Study of Ethical Problems in Medicine and Biomedical and Behavioral Research examined these issues of public concern and has made recommendations for guidance in decision making, institutional policies, and public policy.[1] Its analysis and findings apply to all health professionals and it has stimulated new emphasis on ethical decision making.

Because of the varied subtle ways the patient's hospital experience is controlled by those who work there, physicians and nurses especially, it is useful to explore how others view the ethical questions raised. For example, medical professionals engage in discussions about when to tell patients what is wrong with them or how much information to give to patients about their condition. The nonmedical professional, the ethicist asks, "When, if ever, is it justified to withhold *any* information from a patient about his condition?" Study of this problem of disclosing information to patients has revealed very different perspectives by physicians and patients. In a 1961 study, 88 percent of 208 physicians surveyed said that it is *not* their usual policy to tell patients that they have cancer.[2] On the other hand, a study of 100 cancer patients conducted as early as 1950, found that 89 percent were in favor of physicians telling them they had cancer.[3]

The American Hospital Association and others have developed a Patient's Bill of Rights to encourage active participation by patients in determining their care and treatment. In general, these include the right to be fully informed of one's diagnosis, treatment, and prognosis in terms the layperson can understand. Once this information is provided, the patient or his family should also be told of any possible side effects of treatment, including risks, so that when consent is given, it is truly informed consent. The right to refuse treatment is understood to belong to the patient. Cancer patients in particular have the right to be fully informed about the prognosis of their treatment and should be made aware of treatment alternatives. These patients may come to a decision to discontinue treatment at any point in care, and this should be respected. Patients at the end-stage of disease have the right to be informed of any options for other than hospital care, such as hospice or home care, and should be encouraged to select the site most appropriate for them.

IDENTIFICATION AND REVIEW OF MORAL DILEMMAS

Nurses and others should rationally consider ethical decisions. In this process, it is helpful to use a structure for systematic identification and review of the key elements of a moral dilemma. One writer suggests a three-step process for this identification and review:[4]

1. Develop a data base that provides the information necessary for moral inquiry. For example, what is the problem; who are the people involved in its solution; what are the available choices?
2. Review and consider the questions that deal with decision making—questions regarding the criteria to be used, who the decision makers are, the question of informed consent, and others.
3. Examine and select the ethical theory or theories that apply in each case. For instance, one can approach the dilemma from a utilitarian position, which leads to the choice having the greatest good for the greatest number of people, or from a more traditional medical ethic, which values the individual patient and leads to mobilizing any necessary resources to assist him.

One must also recognize that there are no easy answers to ethical/moral dilemmas, and structures such as this one only guide the questioner through the process.

Ethical Issues in Cancer Care

Some of the more frequently occurring ethical issues in care of patients with cancer are presented in this section. Patients make choices all along the way whether to undergo surgery, radiation, chemotherapy, or other interventions. The practical challenge to nurses and physicians is to fully inform patients, not to consciously manipulate the patient's decision, and to abide by it once it is made.

Nurses feel "in the middle" of many ethical issues. This is certainly so in the case of the physician who does not tell the patient that she has cancer, thinking it the "right" thing to do for the patient. The patient turns her questions about cancer and about what is really wrong with her to the nurse. In another case, the family asks the nurse not to tell their mother she has cancer. What is the nurse to do? Does he or she "follow the doctor's orders"? Where does the nurse stand, and with what support? Yarling reviews just such a dilemma, and challenges the reader further by postulating that though such a decision requires a degree of medical knowledge, it should not be based on medical criteria but rather presents a moral decision based "on the recognition of prevailing rights and obligations."[5]

DECISION NOT TO PROLONG DYING

Nurses caring for cancer patients and their families are very familiar with the point in treatment when either the patient, the family, or the nurse or physician asks, "Is it right to continue treatment?" The answer to this question depends in great part on the questioner, but there are some ethical guidelines to consider. In a statement related to the distinction between ordinary and extraordinary means, Pope Pius XII said:

> But morally one is held to use only ordinary means—according to circumstances of persons, places, times, and cultures—that is to say, means that do not involve any grave burden for oneself or another. A more strict obligation would be too burdensome for most people and would render the attainment of the higher, more important good too difficult. Life, health, all temporal activities are in fact subordinated to spiritual ends. On the other hand, one is not forbidden to take more than the strictly necessary steps to preserve life and health.[6]

The above statement has provided medical care providers with some, but certainly not complete, direction. As technologies advance, the definitions of ordinary and extraordinary change. The question of withdrawing treatment once begun is also part of this question. Robert Veatch points out that ethicists see little difference between starting extraordinary life-sustaining treatments, and stopping them once they are implemented, while physicians are more likely to draw a distinction between the two.[7]

Jewish religious law permits the physician to discontinue any treatment to patients in the end-stage of life which would artificially delay death. Both Jewish and Catholic moral law forbid any form of active intervention to end life. Protestant views are in part more liberal, in theory endorsing passive euthanasia—the deliberate withholding of treatment in order to hasten death.[8]

Regardless of one's religious affiliation, people have ethical perspectives that guide them. In confronting this question of prolonging life, one first seeks out the wish of the patient. In the presence of advanced disease with no hope of recovery and a steady decline in biological function, it is the patient, fully informed, who has the right to decide whether to continue treatment. It is also the right of the patient to determine whether he or she wants to be resuscitated in the event of respiratory or cardiac arrest, as this is the end-point of the treatment continuum.

LIVING WILLS

Consumers and potential patients recognize that they may one day be in a position in which health professionals, known or unknown to them, may make decisions for them. Against this possibility, they execute documents to set forth their wishes for treatment. The Euthanasia Educational Council has drafted a model letter for this purpose, called the "living will":

To my family, my physician, my clergyman, my lawyer: If the time comes when I can no longer take part in decisions for my own future, let this statement stand as the testament of my wishes:

If there is no reasonable expectation of my recovery from physical or mental disability, I, _____, request that I be allowed to die and not be kept alive by artificial means or heroic measures.

Death is as much a reality as birth, growth, maturity, and old age—it is the one certainty. I do not fear death as much as I fear the indignity of deterioration, dependence, and hopeless pain. I ask that medication be mercifully administered to me for terminal suffering even if it hastens the moment of death.

This request is made after careful consideration. Although this document is not legally binding, you who care for me will, I hope, feel morally bound to follow its mandate. I recognize that it places a heavy burden of responsibility upon you, and it is with the intention of sharing that responsibility and of mitigating any feelings of guilt that this statement is made.

(Signed) _____

Date _____

Witnessed by:

_____

The biggest problem with the living will is that it cannot be constructed with enough specificity for all situations that might occur.

The important principle of living wills is to preserve the patient's right to make decisions about his care. One suggestion of an alternative to a living will is a written statement by a competent person that relegates to another of his choice the power of attorney to make decisions regarding medical treatment if he is unable. The power of attorney legally vests authority in the patient's agent if the patient is unable to exercise it.

SUPPORTIVE CARE VS. AGGRESSIVE TREATMENT

Once a decision has been made to not prolong dying, and active treatment is withdrawn, a new set of guidelines is put in place to provide the patient with comfort while the disease proceeds. This very special kind of care is primarily nursing care. The comfort-providing activities of the nurse become paramount. Pain-control becomes a major goal, as well as basic comfort measures such as skin care, nutritional support, and the maintenance of bowel function. The goal is to maintain the patient's comfort using ordinary means, and recognizing the limitations of these measures.

Ethical questions about decisions for the proper use of pain medication frequently occur. The central dilemma concerns the patient's desire to be relieved of the suffering that chronic and severe pain imposes upon him, while avoiding the serious risks that large doses of narcotics present, especially the suppression of neurological and respiratory function. Some apprehension has been expressed by health professionals that the liberal use of narcotics may be interpreted as passive euthanasia, but those who are knowledgeable about the proper use of these drugs in managing extreme pain dispute this concern. Hospice programs have been helpful in developing drug mixtures and administration regimens that prevent the experience of extreme pain. Nurses caring for cancer patients who have pain control as a major problem should properly assess and treat this serious problem. The following statement provides a widely accepted ethical framework for considering approaches to pain control: "It is not euthanasia to give a dying person sedatives and analgesics for the alleviation of pain when such a measure is judged necessary, even though they may deprive the patient of the use of reason, or shorten his life."[9]

Whether caring for the terminally ill patient and his or her family in the hospital or at home, the nurse's goal is the provision of comfort and maintaining the patient as free of pain as possible. Dying patients also find great reassurance in not being left alone, so providing open access to family and friends makes dying in a hospital more tolerable. The concepts put forth by the hospice movement have had a great influence on hospital care of the dying and support for family throughout and after the patient's ordeal. Hospital rules about visiting hours or other limiting practices are not appropriately applied to these patients.

The advances of technology that have brought nurses face to face with complex ethical problems will continue, and probably at an accelerated rate. Nurses must prepare themselves to deal with these complex problems. Nurses working together, confronting similar ethical issues, should take the opportunity to discuss these issues in a formal way, such as in "ethical rounds," and develop their competence in this aspect of patient care.

REFERENCES

1. President's Commission for the Study of Ethical Problems in Medicine and Biomedical and Behavioral Research. Deciding to forgo life-sustaining treatment: Ethical, Medical and Legal issues in treatment decisions. Washington: U.S. Government Printing Office, 1983.

2. **Ioken D.** What to tell cancer patients. JAMA 175:1120, 1961.

3. **Kelly WD and Friesen SR.** Do cancer patients want to be told? SURGERY 27:822, 1950.

4. **Aroskar MA.** Anatomy of an ethical dilemma: The theory. AM J NURS 80:661, 1980.

5. **Yarling RR.** Ethical analysis of a nursing problem: The scope of nursing practice in disclosing the truth to terminal patients. SUPERVISOR NURSE 9:40, May 1978.

6. **Pius XII.** The Pope speaks: Prolongation of life. L'OSSERVATORE ROMANO 4:393, 1957.

7. **Veatch RM.** DEATH, DYING, AND THE BIOLOGICAL REVOLUTION. New Haven, Conn: Yale University Press, 1978.

8. **Benton RG.** DEATH AND DYING: PRINCIPLES AND PRACTICES IN PATIENT CARE. New York: Van Nostrand Reinhold, 1978.

9. **Beauchamp TL and Childress JF.** PRINCIPLES OF BIOMEDICAL ETHICS. New York: Oxford University Press, 1979.

BIBLIOGRAPHY

Fromer MJ. ETHICAL ISSUES IN HEALTH CARE. St Louis: Mosby, 1981.

Levine M. Nursing ethics and the ethical nurse. AM J NURS 77:845, 1977.

Pence G. ETHICAL OPTIONS IN MEDICINE. Oradell, NJ: Medical Economics, 1980.

Storck JL. Consumer rights and health care. NAC 4:110, 1980.

14

SELECTION OF THE CARE SETTING FOR THE TERMINALLY ILL

PATRICIA M. WALL, RN, BS

New emphasis is being given to the patient and his or her family when the patient requires terminal care. Public interest has stimulated the development of hospice programs and facilities in every part of the country. Hospice is derived from the Latin word *hospitium*, meaning hospitality. In medieval times, religious orders opened their doors to weary pilgrims and travelers. These included not only the hearty and strong but also the sick, the dying, and those members of society who could not care for themselves. The monks and nuns provided care and comfort until their guests were able to continue on their journey. Hospice, hospitality, hotel, and, more recently, hospital have come to suggest a generosity of spirit rendered to those who come your way.

Gradually, hospice came to be identified with the special care given to sick and dying people. The Irish Sisters of Charity opened Our Lady's Hospice in Dublin in 1846 and St. Joseph's Hospice in London in 1905. More recently, the impetus and inspiration for hospice has come from England. Through the work of Dr. Cicely Saunders, director of St. Christopher's Hospice in London, and her colleagues, hospice has come to mean excellence of care for the terminally ill, embracing the many specialities of the health-care professions. Doctors, pharmacologists, nurses, social workers, clergymen, music therapists, artists, and others have joined in an unprecedented fashion to discover ways to enhance the quality of life for people faced with a terminal illness.

Hospice has flourished most readily in those countries where national health-care systems exist, notably in England and Canada. St. Christopher's Hospice in London and the Palliative Care Service of the Royal Victoria Hospital (RVH) in Montreal continue to be in the vanguard of the hospice movement. They both have extensive research and educational programs designed to promote the hospice concept. To palliate is "to reduce the violence of; abate." In the hospice context, it means the relief of pain and other troubling symptoms. This term can be considered to be synonymous with hospice care. The PCS, through its affiliation with the McGill University Medical School, conducts research for new ways to alleviate both the physical and psychological pain many terminally ill people experience. The PCS exists as a facility to care for dying patients, as a service to the RVH to meet the needs of patients dying in other wards of the hospital, as a home-care program for patients admitted to its service who prefer to die at home, and as a research and teaching arm of McGill University. The PCS offers continuing-education programs and internship experiences in its facility.

The Hospice of Marin in Marin County, California; Hospice Inc. of New Haven, Connecticut; and the hospice team at St. Luke's Hospital in New York City are pioneers in the development of the hospice movement in this country. The National Hospice Organization in McLean, Virginia, has identified standards of care for hospices. As insurance company coverage of hospice care and federal funding become more available, hospice will increasingly become an integral part of our health-care system.

The implementation of the hospice concept in this country has taken many forms. A hospice may exist as a unit within an acute-care institution; as a service within an acute-care institution, having residential, ambulatory, and home-care patients; or as an organization of volunteers offering home care. Some hospices are free-standing facilities offering residential care and have no hospital affiliation. Some extended-care facilities and nursing homes have developed hospice programs. In many states, there are organizations that act as clearinghouses for information, education, staff training, and publicity.

Patient Considerations

The need to plan for the patient's care when death is inevitable can be very upsetting to the patient and his or her family. Plans and dreams must be reassessed. The selection of the caring facility depends on the attitudes of the patient and family about where the patient wants to die and the resources available to accommodate that wish. It also depends on the patient's physician and their mutual hopes and expectations regarding the patient's prognosis. The patient's physical condition and the care required to maintain complex treatment measures that have been initiated, such as a tracheostomy, feeding tubes, or an ostomy, also influence selection of the care setting. Whether the family is able to manage the equipment used for supportive care at home or can afford nursing care are important considerations. Selection of the care site is also determined by the availability of care services either within the acute-care institution or elsewhere in the community in which the patient lives.

CONTINUITY OF CARE

In many instances, the hospital in which the patient has received oncology care has a hospice or terminal-care program that allows for continuity of care. The hospice team is introduced to the patient who needs hospice care while active therapy is being administered. Involvement of the hospice team in consultation with the oncology team promotes quality-of-life measures to meet the spiritual and bodily needs of the patient.

When active treatment is no longer advisable, the transfer of the patient to the hospice team is then easier for the patient, family, and care givers. The nursing-care plan implemented during the acute phase is continued, with appropriate adjustment to meet the changing needs of the patient in the terminal phase of care.

In a hospital that does not have an organized hospice program, the health-care team responsible for providing care during the aggressive phase of treatment also plans for terminal care. The transition from aggressive therapy to terminal care is more difficult to plan if organized services are not available. When the option of hospice care is not available, treatment may be continued until the moment of death. Nurses must then be available to patients on two levels. On one level, they must support the patient in his effort to fight and survive cancer; on another level, they must accept the possibility of death. A delicate balance between hope and trust and acceptance of whatever may happen is required in these situations.

PLANNING CARE

The planning of nursing care for the terminal phases of illness can challenge your creativity. You must resolve personal feelings about the patient's inevitable death and must remain an objective, concerned member of the health-care team during this phase. Caring is demonstrated by activities such as compiling a list of favorite foods the patient loves or asking the hospital librarian to find long-cherished books or poems the patient would like to read or hear. You can find quiet times for the patient to use a tape recorder to record his thoughts as a memento for loved ones.

Planning nursing care for the dying patient may be guided by the following recommendations:

1. Keep the patient's remaining days free of distressing symptoms.
2. Simplify all care of the patient. Eliminate intricate and complicated procedures.
3. Ensure physical and spiritual comfort.
4. Enable the patient to resolve business concerns and enjoy personal relationships to the fullest measure possible.

Many of the treatments used to ameliorate symptoms require hospitalization in the acute-care setting. Such procedures as placement of a gastrostomy tube, surgical intervention to relieve pain, and titration of narcotic analgesics require medical and nursing supervision in the acute-care setting. You must then provide "hospice" care to patients and their families, even when such a program does not exist within the institution.

STAGES OF GRIEF

One of your most frustrating experiences can be observing the dying patient and family await death. Elisabeth Kubler-Ross described stages of death: denial and isolation, anger, bargaining, depression, and acceptance. The transition from one stage to another is seldom direct. There may be reversal and repetition, and the patient and family may never be at the same stage at the same time.

Other researchers have disputed the clinical application of Kubler-Ross's stages of death and have found that dying patients experience a wide variety of psychologic responses during dying. The theories, although controversial, may help you understand the needs of dying patients and the complexities of assessing them.

Assessment of denial can be especially perplexing. Denial may be complete—that is, the patient refuses to consider the inevitable; this denial may be transitional or reversible. Or the denial may be partial—that is, the patient may accept some aspects of the consequences of the disease but not others. The patient may also be selective in denial. An example is a woman who was quite knowledgeable about her condition. She elected to undergo some therapy, but put limits on how extensive the therapy should be. Her husband, however, could not come to grips with her declining health. She recognized his feelings and in his presence displayed an air of indifference regarding her prognosis. She attempted to preserve their relationship as he struggled with the dilemma of her impending death. But with health-care team members, she acknowledged her impending death. It was her way of coping, of controlling her environment, of planning her remaining days. As illustrated by this patient's experience, a nursing assessment of patient denial is difficult to make and should be done with great care and after several observations.

Another aspect of daily life that the nurse must be mindful of is the tendency to be future-oriented. The most casual of comments implies a future dimension. Blithe remarks, such as "Have a good night" or "I'll take care of you next week when I'm back," are not free of ironically dire implications for the patient who knows he will soon die.

Family Needs

During the terminal phase, some form of acute care is often required for patient maintenance. Certain elements in the acute-care setting can promote a caring environment. Many patients and their families wish to attempt every life-saving therapy possible. Others wish only to ensure the patient's physical comfort and emotional peace. The varying preferences of patients and their families can be accommodated in the acute-care setting. Many families prefer private rooms for the patient's care, and whenever possible that request should be met. Having food or kitchen equipment available allows families to bring and heat favorite foods for the patient. Family members may wish to stay with their loved one through the night. Cots can be made available for that purpose.

Every effort should be made to assist the patient and family achieve their goals. People die as they have lived, and family relationships are not always harmonious. Conflicts often are exacerbated by illness and impending death of a family member. Attempt to determine how both patient and family needs can best be met and make an effort to ensure that the various resources of the hospital are available to patients. The social worker, and both the hospital chaplain and the family's own clergy and other health-care professionals may be intimately involved with the patient and family during the terminal days and during the bereavement period. Often the coordination of all these care givers is up to you.

THE DEATH
The nurse is often the first person to meet a family member at the actual death of a loved one. If the family was not present when the patient died, family members may ask the nurse for details of the death. When? How? What happened? What was done for the patient? The way in which you respond to these questions has a great effect on the way family members integrate news of the patient's death. A calm, simple description of the events leading up to the death will allay fears of the family; knowing that everything possible was done for the patient is comforting. Whether or not the death was anticipated, the actual death is always a shock for family and nurse alike. Before making subjective comments about the patient, listen for cues from the family and attempt to determine what their immediate concerns are. Praising family members for the care and support they gave the patient, staying with the family, and helping them organize their thoughts and begin necessary funeral arrangements are also helpful.

BEREAVEMENT CARE
Bereavement care begins at the moment of death. Families who have endured a lengthy course of illness with their loved one frequently have close relationships with the nursing staff. Nurses, too, often feel the immediate loss of a patient and family. Often there are no mechanisms to complete the relationship, and yet many families and the nurses who cared for them feel a need to accomplish closure. One device to complete the nurse-family relationship is a bereavement letter you can send to the key survivor of the patient. It gives you an opportunity to acknowledge the death of the patient and to commend the survivors for the care they extended to the patient. Nurses often meet families who experience tremendous burdens while managing the care of their loved ones. This family devotion needs to be recognized. The bereavement letter can praise families and also acknowledge the distress and concerns the survivors may have following the patient's death. A feeling of numbness, loss of appetite, inability to concentrate, a yearning for the lost person are just a few of the symptoms the grievers may experience. They need to know that for a reasonable period of time these changes and stresses are quite normal and will gradually dissipate. The bereavement letter provides an opportunity for the survivor to then return a gesture of gratitude to the nursing staff and other care givers.

A bereavement letter is one thing to think about and quite another to write. When one has trouble beginning the letter, which often occurs, it's useful to imagine meeting the person on the street. What would you say then? This exercise helps to write the first line. The following points may be helpful in composing the rest of a bereavement letter:

- send the letter to the key person in the patient's life;
- send the letter from two weeks to two months following the death;
- offer condolences, sympathy, sorrow, and express sadness;
- recall the struggle the patient experienced;
- in a positive way, mention the role the key person played in the care of the loved one;
- describe a special experience you shared with the patient;
- comment on how difficult the adjustment must be for the survivor;
- mention the potential for cherished memories of the loved one.

All of the above points are seldom incorporated into one letter, but all of the items may be useful on one occasion or another.

MEMORIAL SERVICES
Some nurses find it rewarding to attend funeral services of a patient they have cared for. Staffing schedules can be adjusted to permit nurses to do this. Another avenue to aid in the grieving process is a memorial service in the hospital chapel. Services can be held on a regular basis, every two or three months. Family members and friends of patients who have died in the hospital during the previous period can be invited. Relatives of nononcology patients would appreciate being included on the guest list, as they have similar needs and stresses during bereavement. The service can be conducted by the hospital chaplain or a clergyman from the community served by the hospital. Nurses and other health-care givers may wish to participate in the memorial service.

HOSPICE AND HOME CARE
For the patient and his family who prefer home care rather than institutional care, community hospice programs conducted by Visiting Nurses' Associations (VNA) or similar agencies can provide care. In these programs, a nurse discharge planner and primary nurses may assist patients and their families in making arrangements for patients who desire home hospice care. The patient's primary nurse outlines the specific nursing care needs. The patient's attending physician prescribes medications and other necessary treatment to promote the comfort of the patient. The discharge planner or primary nurse communicates this information to the hospice coordinator who meets with the patient

either in the hospital before discharge or later at the patient's home to make an initial assessment of patient and family needs.

The full range of services provided by the agency—social services, nursing, nutrition, and physical therapy—can be made available. Financial arrangements vary and are often based on the patient's ability to pay. In some communities, there is a volunteer hospice corps, and a volunteer may be assigned to the family.

Nursing homes also can provide the specialized care a dying patient, particularly an oncology patient, may need. When family resources are exhausted and patient care becomes too difficult for the family to manage, they may use nursing-home care.

Community services, such as the VNA, may be used during the treatment phase of cancer diseases and, consequently, many patients admitted to their hospice service are already known to the nursing staff. Continuity in the care provided is important to the patient and family because it offers stability in a time of crisis.

Some hospice programs are primarily an organization of volunteers, many of whom may be health-care professionals. These hospice programs often have no headquarters but operate on a network basis with the patient at home. An example is the Hospice of the North Shore, near Chicago. Families living in the suburbs in this area may turn to the hospice for care and support. The hospice admits patients with less than a six-month expected life span. They have found that longer involvement with a patient can interfere with the business of living, and their service may become a source of conflict rather than the support that is intended. A sufficient length of time is needed, however, to develop a helpful relationship with the patient and family.

Patient referral to the hospice may be made by the doctor, primary nurse, or a family member. In fact, some hospice programs receive the majority of referrals from families of dying patients. When the request is received, the patient care coordinator of the hospice meets with the patient, either in the hospital or in the patient's home, makes an initial assessment of patient and family needs, and describes what the hospice can offer. If indicated in this initial contact with the patient, a VNA may be requested to make a nursing assessment of the patient's care needs. The VNA may or may not provide care, depending on a mutual decision made by the family, the hospice, and the VNA. The hospice assigns volunteers to the patient. They perform myriad tasks, from running errands to reading to the patient to keeping a vigil with the patient while family members take a rest. Volunteers are usually required to donate five hours a week to their assigned family. Should the patient's deteriorating condition require readmission to the hospital, the volunteers frequently continue their contacts with the patient and family in the hospital.

A summary of patient care provided by the hospice, which accompanies the patient on readmission to the hospital, is useful to promote continuity of care. The summary is similar to a continuity of care form or discharge plan used by the primary nurse when discharging patients to the VNA or nursing homes. It should describe the measures that have contributed to the patient's peace of mind and general well-being, up-to-date information on family dynamics, and list other persons, such as relatives and clergy, who have been a source of support to the patient. This information could then be incorporated into the nursing care plan for the patient.

The volunteers of the hospice often continue contact with their assigned family following the death of the patient. They may help with the funeral arrangements or continue to perform the tasks they had been doing. Their presence helps mitigate the sense of loss experienced by grieving people. It's not unusual for volunteer contacts to continue up to a year following the patient's death.

The Hospice of the North Shore has made a major contribution to the quality of life for many people. A continuing concern of the hospice is the consistency of its referring network. They stress community education and have an active speakers bureau. As the community becomes better informed about their services, timely referrals may result. Three to four weeks, they have found, is the optimum time to offer supportive care to a patient and his family. Requests made less than a week before the patient dies often result in only perfunctory care. It simply takes more than a week to thoroughly assess a given situation and provide specialized care. In some instances, hospice personnel provide education for the hospital's nursing and medical staff members to make them aware of their services and to encourage referrals from the hospital before a patient is on his death bed.

SUMMARY

When it becomes apparent that aggressive therapy is no longer appropriate for the cancer patient, planning must be directed toward terminal care. Such care, often referred to as hospice care, is usually a responsibility of the primary nurse in the acute-care hospital. By choice or happenstance, some patients will die in the acute-care setting. The nurse must assess both the needs of the patient and of the family during the terminal phase. With a successful plan of care, the nurse can help the patient and family spend their final days together in an atmosphere of peace and serenity.

BIBLIOGRAPHY

Ajemian I and Mount BM (eds). THE RVH MANUAL ON PALLIA-TIVE/HOSPICE CARE. New York: Arno, 1980.

Kubler-Ross E. ON DEATH AND DYING. New York:Macmillan, 1969.

Parkes CM. BEREAVEMENT: STUDIES OF GRIEF IN ADULT LIFE. New York: Pelican, 1975.

Pattison EM. The living-dying process. In PSYCHOSOCIAL CARE OF THE DYING PATIENT, Garfield CA (ed). New York: McGraw-Hill, 1978.

Roberts L. Drugs in the palliative care of the cancer patient and emotional aspects of the cancer illness. In PALLIATIVE CARE OF THE CANCER PATIENT, Hickey RC (ed). Boston: Little, Brown, 1967.

Saunders C. Hospice care. In THE RVH MANUAL ON PALLIATIVE/HOSPICE CARE. New York: Arno, 1980.

Ufema J. Grieving families. NURSING 81, 11:81, Nov 1981.

Weisman AD. THE REALIZATION OF DEATH. New York: Jason Aronson, 1974.

15

THE END STAGE OF CANCER

JUNE WERNER, RN, MSN, CNAA

Weisman contends that some deaths are better than others.[1] Three major categories of information helpful in assessing any patient's potential for a good death are disease, personality, and social context. The category of social context refers to significance of relationships, role of work, stability of finances, importance of religion, and role of family. Your ability to successfully meet the patient's and the family's assessed needs depends on your clinical competence, the capacity to be supportive, being a caring human being, and on a support system readily available to you.

An important nursing role is supporting patients and families as death approaches. Patients who have end-stage cancer may be cared for either in the hospital or at home. Those who spend their last days in the hospital do so either because their condition is so complicated that they cannot be cared for at home, or because the family members are so overwhelmed that they cannot provide care in the home. In either case, the patient and the family endure similar problems, are vulnerable, and often weary from continuous coping. In almost every instance, a humane and caring environment sustains the patient and the family.

Whether the patient is hospitalized or at home, the two major areas of nursing care are provision of physical care and comfort for the patient and support and care of the family. Nurses who have had a sustained relationship with the patient and family during earlier phases of care can be of particular help to the patient and family during life's end stage. Nurses who have gained the patient's and the family's trust and confidence through previous contacts can better maintain communication necessary for effective care of the dying patient, often finding a great sense of purpose in participating with patients and families as they negotiate this stage of life.

The nursing process used in care of patients in previous phases of illness continues as the patient enters the end stage of life. Use of the nursing process ensures continuity. Assessment, planning, and implementation keep the patient feeling secure and free from pain. Evaluation of the dying patient provides information that can be used to improve the care of other patients. Just as important as the nursing process and the therapeutic measures is the climate you can provide to sustain the quality of the patient's life and that of the family during this time.

Your effectiveness in caring for the dying patient depends on whether you come to terms with the roles of counselor and care giver. Frequently, one hears or reads that in order to be helpful to the dying, the helping professionals must have come to terms with their own death. Experience will tell that this is not entirely true, although nurses may learn something about coping with or anticipating their own death by being involved in the care of their patients. With appropriate support, nurses can learn to be effective in the supportive care of patients in end-stage cancer. Through experience you learn that death is not easy to explain and that each person's death, even if expected, stimulates highly individualized responses in the patient, family members, and care givers. Recognition of the varied responses to death is perhaps more important for one's roles as counselor and care giver than it is for facing one's own death.

Physical Care and Comfort

Physical care and comfort for the patient are major areas of nursing for the dying patient. Effective physical care of terminal patients can greatly contribute to a peaceful death. Whether the patient is in the hospital or at home, the care needs are similar. Nursing care of the terminally ill patient is predicated on the patient's perception of his or her needs, which are more important than the perceptions that others may have.

Many patient needs have been described in detail in earlier chapters of this book. Some emphasized in care of the dying patient are briefly described below. They include pain management and relaxation; control of constipation, nausea, vomiting; adequate nutrition; and prevention of decubiti.

PAIN MANAGEMENT

Intractable pain in the patient with advanced cancer presents one of the greatest nursing challenges. The technology of pain management has increased through efforts of professionals in pain centers, pharmaceutical laboratories, and hospices throughout the country. Advances in prescribing medications and ways of administering medications that are effective for patients in acute distress have improved the capability to manage pain. You may find it helpful to assist the patient in keeping a diary in which he or she can record the medications given, the effects of the medications, and the symptoms experienced prior to taking medications. Review of the diary gives the patient and family an opportunity to observe the time frames in which the patient becomes uncomfortable and the amount of time it takes for medication to provide relief.

It is essential that you evaluate the effectiveness of pain medication. Your assessment can provide information the physician needs to prescribe the most effective combination of medications. The therapeutic effect of narcotics can be enhanced, for example, by medications that relieve anxiety if in your assessment the patient has a high level of anxiety. Nursing measures may also be initiated to enhance the therapeutic effect of pain-relieving medications.

When the terminal cancer patient is cared for at home, the family must be taught to administer the medication and to assess the patient's response to that medication to provide the physician with the information needed to adjust dosage, if necessary. Ineffective pain management at home is often the reason for readmitting the patient to the hospital. If the patient and family wish the patient to remain at home, an investment in time and energy in learning to manage the patient's pain is essential. The nurse may initially teach the patient's family members the necessary care measures while the patient is in the hospital, with follow-up home visits to help them learn to give care. Teaching the family member to keep an ongoing record of the time of onset of discomfort, time of administration of the medication or other therapeutic measures, and time of beginning of relief of pain will help in their evaluation of the effectiveness of care. Positive reinforcement of the family members' contribution to pain management often gives them the strength to continue care as the patient nears death.

Relaxation techniques are also helpful measures for patients with pain. Deep breathing exercises, muscle relaxation exercises, imagery, or meditation may help the patient tolerate pain. When conventional and noninvasive methods of treating intractable pain fail, surgical intervention to interrupt the pain pathway may be necessary, as described in Chapter 11.

CONSTIPATION

Patients with terminal cancer may suffer great discomfort because of constipation. The resulting distention, the pressure of the distended abdomen on the diaphragm, and the accompanying flatulence compound the patient's pain and discomfort. A plan should be established in the hospital to help the family learn the measures most helpful to the particular patient. Prune juice or strained fruit at bedtime or commercial strained baby fruit can be used in the hospital or at home. The family should be taught the necessary procedures, including enemas and the removal of fecal impactions. A public health nurse or visiting nurse can provide this care if the family is unable to do so.

NAUSEA AND VOMITING

Nausea and vomiting can plague the terminal cancer patient. They can be managed by the careful selection of foods, by small frequent feedings and often by prescribed medication, given by suppository. These medications should be given on a carefully regulated schedule, when necessary, to prevent nausea and vomiting.

NUTRITION

Terminal patients are characteristically anorexic. They are often not interested in food and even the smell of food makes some patients feel nauseated. As described in Chapter 10, special nutrition formulas are available. Patients at this stage can have anything they really enjoy and feel comfortable eating. Patients, when asked what they would really like to have, sometimes identify a food from childhood—a ginger cookie, Indian pudding, fresh lemonade. Such patients may not eat a great deal of anything, but a few spoonfuls of something they really enjoy and can tolerate is a blessing.

If possible, the patient should be sufficiently hydrated to prevent the necessity for intravenous fluids. Small, frequent sips of fluids the patient enjoys, given at an agreeable temperature, may be helpful in preventing dehydration.

THE PREVENTION OF DECUBITI

Patients in the end stage of a malignant disease have all the prodromal signs of decubiti, if not actual bedsores. They tend to be bedridden, inadequately nourished, are often dehydrated, and are resistant to moving because they want to remain in a position in which they are most comfortable. For all these reasons, they can develop decubiti, which may make them even more uncomfortable. It is essential to avoid that state. For patients at home, it is very important that the persons taking care of them have been taught how to bathe and turn them and how to use an egg crate mattress or other appropriate device to avoid constant pressure on any one area. The family needs to be taught to assess indications of oncoming decubiti. If treatment is necessary, the family needs to understand the reasons for treatment and be taught by a qualified nurse how to give the treatment correctly.

Comfort and Support

Comfort and support are traditional nursing functions. According to Weisman, an appropriate death presumes good care and management by others.[1] To the extent that he or she has built an effective relationship with the patient, the nurse can be useful to the patient when he is near death.

KNOWLEDGE OF IMPENDING DEATH

The nurse who has cared for a patient over the course of an illness has, it is hoped, developed a relationship with him based on trust and confidence. The nurse who knows the patient can identify patterns in the patient's responses and can provide a climate that fosters open expression of feelings about impending death. Even patients who have been denied the information from physician or family that their illness is terminal usually are aware of impending death. You can be a bridge between the patient and physician or family to reduce ambiguity about the last stages of life. You can document on the chart for the physician why you believe the patient knows he is going to die, and you can share this information in an appropriate way with the family so there are no unsaid words between family and the patient. Once the reality has been established for the patient and for the family with affirmation by the physician, it becomes easier to deal with the presenting problems associated with the patient's death.

EMOTIONAL RESPONSES

Often patients in the end stage of cancer exhibit some form of anger, sometimes even rage. The behavior that rises out of this understandable anger may sap the patients' strength and alienate the people they need most—family and care givers. The patient may be abusive or aggressive, expressing in behavior what he can neither accept nor verbalize.

You can help the patient identify the feelings as anger to help him pass through this phase of his responses. "You seem angry, Mr. Jones. I can understand why you could be. Do you feel angry?" The question gently put may open flood tides of rage and despair. You must be prepared for tears and even a verbal tirade, must stay with the patient while he exhibits this emotional "retention with overflow," perhaps saying nothing but behaving with utmost acceptance. This "event" in the course of the patient's response usually helps to attain some level of acceptance.

If the family members have been exposed to outbursts of anger, abuse, and aggression that they do not understand, you can help by explaining to them that the patient might be angry rather than depressed at what is happening to him. It may be useful to offer the family the comfort of knowing that anger is a usual coping mechanism in patients and to tell them, "We try to help the patient express it so that he 'gets it out of his system.' This expression often makes the patient feel better or become more relaxed."

The goal of the nurse is to comfort both patient and family and to be a bridge of understanding between them throughout this difficult time. Some patients exhibit no anger, but may show signs of various levels of depression. Rare is the person who seems to accept his or her own impending death without some form of resistance. Anger or depression or both in some form can be expected. Like any other crisis the patient experiences, you can manage it so that it becomes productive in improving the quality of the patient's life.

An effective nurse is a very good listener. Active listening is comprehending not only what is said, but also attending to how it is said. An important function of the nurse is not only to talk to or with the patient, but to make it possible for the patient to express concerns, problems, fears, and anxieties at any given time. The question, "What is bothering you most right now?" may be similar to removing the top of a pressure cooker. The patient may be able to ventilate his feelings, may be able to cry, may be able to express thoughts and feelings that have not been formulated up to that point.

You gain information in these sessions. Your responsibility, then, is to act on the patient's concerns. The plan of action may include providing information to the family or to the physician. There may be something you can do for the patient that he has not asked anyone else. A nonreligious man may suddenly want to see his clergyman. A parent who has been alienated from a child over the years may want to see that child. An anniversary or a birthday may need to be celebrated. Or the patient may need to know that indeed he may go home to die rather than to die in the institution.

Keeping the channels of communication open with the patient may mean that you will receive information coming through those channels that is difficult to hear or difficult to resolve. However, the alternative of not giving the patient the opportunity to express his concerns, is unacceptable.

THE NURSE AS COUNSELOR

Burkhalter and Donley feel "the nurse/counselor needs to experience a sense of commitment to assisting the oncology patient to achieve or retain a quality of living regardless of treatment outcomes or probabilities."[2] In the context of counseling, they discuss the characteristics of empathy, attentiveness, honesty, and warmth as necessary for the nurse/counselor. The exercise of these characteristics may place a burden on a nurse caring for this patient; thus, a support system for the nurse is essential. The alternative is to do the tasks of patient care and to avoid making an assessment that would yield information about emotional needs, problems, and unspoken issues on the part of the patient, which can be met only by the nurse acting as a human being.

Nonverbal communication is often more important than any verbal communication at this stage of the patient's illness. A sensitive nurse can see by the expression on the patient's face how he feels, can pick up the subliminal clues that indicate fear, anxiety, or a need to be comforted. The best comfort may be touching the patient, rubbing his back, holding his hand, or simply being there for him, taking 10 minutes to sit beside his bed, while he waits for his family to come. Often the fear of facing impending death alone is the most overwhelming fear patients have. The nurse who has developed the talent for nurturing experiences the greatest rewards from caring for a patient and family in these circumstances.

Hampe's small-scale study on the needs of the grieving spouse in a hospital setting identified eight needs of the family member whose spouse is dying.[3] The needs fall into two categories:

1. There are needs that center on the spouse's relations with the dying patient:
   - to be with the dying person;
   - to feel helpful to the dying person;
   - to be kept informed of the dying person's condition; and
   - to be aware of the dying person's impending death.

2. There are needs that center on the grieving spouse;
- to ventilate his emotions;
- to receive comfort and support from family members; and
- to receive support and comfort from the health professionals.

A concerned nurse is in an excellent position to accommodate these human needs.

FAMILY CARE AND SUPPORT

The psychological impact of the patient with cancer tends to be reflected within the family. A supportive nurse can help family members in the same way he or she assists a patient. For example, family members may exhibit the same kind of behavior normally seen with any human being who is under stress. As the patient advances toward death, communication becomes a problem for the family and for the patient. The stage of hopelessness before acceptance, if indeed acceptance ever comes, is the most difficult time for most families.

The nurses caring for the patient can make assessments and plans, implement those plans, and evaluate their effectiveness related to the needs of the immediate family. It may be appropriate to involve clergymen or social workers in supporting a family. It is often the nurse who identifies the family's need for support and who secures it for them. If the family has an abiding relationship with a clergyman, he can be a great comfort to them. A family that has no clergyman may develop a relationship with a hospital chaplain at this last stage of the patient's illness. A dear friend of the family can also become a precious resource at this time. The nurse must make sure that such a valuable person receives the same extended hospital visiting privileges that family members are accorded.

STAFF NEEDS FOR CARE

Nurses expected to provide a humane and caring environment for patients and their families in the end stage of cancer work in a stressful environment, and support for them is essential. Formal sessions held for nurses taking care of even one patient with cancer, in which they share their feelings and their responses, can be very helpful. Nurses are not spared the sadness of a life coming to an end, particularly in a patient who ordinarily would not be ready to die. Young parents with families, young people, those who may be near the age of the nurses, and "beautiful people" who, at any age, leave the earth impoverished by their absence are examples of patients who may cause an emotional drain on nurses caring for them. Inherent in the effective care of such patients, however, is the possibility of great rewards. Success in this work may expand the nurses' human experience in ways that will contribute to their own lives, deepen their personal wellspring, and contribute to maturity.

In some settings, a psychiatric nurse is assigned to patient care units as a resource person, helping with the support of the staff on a formal ongoing basis, meeting with them regularly as long as needed. The purposes of such meetings are:

- to ventilate and express feelings related to caring for the dying cancer patient;
- to develop a trusting, open support system that acts as a cushion for stress that can be experienced in oncology nursing; and
- to foster problem-solving techniques when particular patient problems arise.

The resource nurse may also act as a consultant to the nurses to help them find better ways to intervene on behalf of patients and family having difficulties. A social worker may also be a very good resource person under these circumstances.

In any case, it's counterproductive for nurses to provide care to cancer patients without some means to express their feelings to and with each other and to gain support from the group. In metropolitan and rural areas, the American Cancer Society can be contacted to locate resource people who might present programs or work with nursing staff in support groups or consultation.

After Death

Better anticipatory coping, less distress, fewer unresolved problems, more support, and more complete preparation make a better death, which, in turn, evokes a better bereavement. The preliminary procedures take the edge off dismay, and horror out of actual loss, and subsequently lead to milder mourning. A better quality of care before death contributes to a better climate for bereavement. But even when the death has been anticipated and the family is relieved that the patient will no longer suffer, death creates a crisis for the family, and nursing intervention is needed to help the family cope with the loss.

The emergence of hospices has not only greatly improved the care of terminally ill patients, but also has enhanced recognition of the importance of care of the family after the death of the patient. Some hospices provide volunteers to work with the patient and family. After death, a volunteer keeps in touch with the family through the funeral and afterwards if necessary.

Families may have great needs for care following a death. Some families have a very difficult time coping. The death and the stress that accompanies loss and grief can cause family members to become ill, or at least exhibit maladaptive behavior. In such cases, bereavement counseling is now available through community agencies or clergymen and in some hospice programs.

Nurses can be helpful to families after death by being there for them, by giving them a comfortable climate in which to cry or talk. Thinking and talking about death need not be morbid; such activities may be quite the opposite. Ignorance and fear of death cast a shadow over life. Knowing about and accepting death erases this shadow and makes life freer of fears and anxieties. The fuller and richer people's experience of life, the less death seems to matter to them. Education for death is a major task in our time and culture. Basically, it is education for life and should be an underlying feature in all educational programs, schools, and throughout the media.

The opportunity for the patient who is dying to be attended by the people he loves—by the family—eases the acceptance of the reality of loss, which is one of the major tasks of mourning. Attending someone at the moment of death is anxiety-producing. Families tend to fear this experience. The nurse, comforting, secure, engendering strength, may help to make it an experience that allows for closeness and comfort.

Families must have the opportunity to express their immediate emotion—to cry, to withdraw, to be together, unhurried. They need privacy and time. You can provide a climate of trust in which this can take place. If you have had a sustained relationship with a family in which the patient has died, you may attend the funeral and keep in touch with that family for some time after the death.

FAMILY REINTEGRATION

The first task of the family is to mourn. Those who can't mourn, who deny their grief, may need some professional help. The unresolved grief impacts on the health and well-being of those who suffer from it. Most bereaved people, however, return to a normal life without therapeutic help after they have mourned their loved one in whatever way or however long was appropriate to them. If you keep in touch with families you may observe the reintegration of families, the closing of ranks, the adaptation of roles, or sometimes the pathology that results not so much from the death, but from the family's response to that death.

Nurses who have participated in the support of a patient who has had a good death may remember it as an inspirational experience. Nursing is one of the few professions that affords its practitioners experience of some modeling in dying. Obviously, this has the possibility of making a contribution to the life of the nurse.

REFERENCES

1. **Weisman AD.** COPING WITH CANCER. New York: McGraw-Hill, 1979.
2. **Burkhalter PK and Donley DL (eds).** DYNAMICS OF ONCOLOGY NURSING. New York: McGraw-Hill, 1978.
3. **Hampe SO.** Needs of the grieving spouse in a hospital setting. NURS RES 24:113, 1975.

BIBLIOGRAPHY

Forsyth DM. The hardest job of all. NURSING 82, 12:82, 1982.

Germain, C. THE CANCER UNIT: AN ETHNOGRAPHY. Wakefield, Mass: Nursing Resources, 1979.

Martin A. How to help when a patient goes home to die. NURS LIFE 2:671, 1981.

TOWARD A GENTLER DYING. Baltimore: Church Hospital, 1981.

Williams CA. Role considerations in care of the dying patient. IMAGE 14:8, 1982.

BIBLIOGRAPHY FOR PATIENTS' FAMILIES

Grollman EA. CONCERNING DEATH. Boston: Beacon, 1974.

————. EXPLAINING DEATH TO CHILDREN. Boston: Beacon, 1969.

————. TALKING ABOUT DEATH. Boston: Beacon, 1976.

————. WHEN YOUR LOVED ONE IS DYING. Boston: Beacon, 1980.

Pincus L. DEATH AND THE FAMILY: THE IMPORTANCE OF MOURNING. New York: Random House, 1976.

INDEX

RN Nursing Assessment Series
  The Well Adult
  ISBN 0-87489-281-3

  Respiratory Problems
  ISBN 0-87489-282-1

  Metabolic Problems
  ISBN 0-87489-284-8

  Gastrointestinal Problems
  ISBN 0-87489-285-6

  Genitourinary Problems
  ISBN 0-87489-286-4

  Neurologic Problems
  ISBN 0-87489-287-2

  Musculoskeletal Problems
  ISBN 0-87489-288-0

  Cardiovascular Problems
  ISBN 0-87489-289-9

  The Well Infant and Child
  ISBN 0-87489-290-2

RN's Survival Sourcebook: Coping With Stress
Gloria Ferraro Donnelly, R.N., M.S.N.
ISBN 0-87489-299-6

RN's Sex Q & A: Candid Advice for You and Your Patients
Dorothy DeMoya, R.N., M.S.N., Armando DeMoya, M.D., and
Howard Lewis
ISBN 0-87489-360-7

For information, write to:
MEDICAL ECONOMICS BOOKS
Oradell, New Jersey 07649
Or dial toll-free: 1-800-223-0581, ext. 2755
(Within the 201 area: 262-3030, ext. 2755)